Mary is an experienced Homeopath who has now written this excellent text. She draws on her deep knowledge of Homeopathy, and her many years of treating patients, as a way to heal. The book is suffused with the essence of Homeopathic philosophy combined with insights from her own practice. I can thoroughly recommend this book for anyone interested in the true meaning of health and how Homeopathy can help us attain it.

Dr Stephen Gascoigne, medical doctor, acupuncturist, herbalist, author of *The Prescribed Drug Guide: A Holistic Perspective*

A very well written book. A must-read for everybody who intends to know what Homeopathy is all about. Very simple to understand and a delight to read. Her remedy indications with tips are worth remembering.

Dr Farokh J Master MD(Hom), author of *The Homeopathic Dream Dictionary*

A Little at a Time is a charming little book! A highly readable introduction to the kinds of healing possible with Homeopathy, it covers all the basics. It includes interesting anecdotes, advice on remedies for self-help situations, and lots of good advice on healthy living in general. It's a great book for the curious person who knows that "all is not well" with conventional health care and is intrigued by what Homeopathy may have to offer.

Amy L Lansky PhD, author of *Impossible Cure: The Promise of Homeopathy* and *Active Consciousness: Awakening the Power Within*

Mary English has given us an excellent introductory book on Homeopathy. She explains the basic principles clearly and concisely but with enough background to add some depth of understanding. The reader can begin at once to prescribe for everyday problems, while understanding when professional help is needed. Written in a friendly, conversational tone, this book is a pleasure to read.

Alan V Schmukler, editor of *Homeopathy 4 Everyone*

Mary has written a great introduction to Homeopathy. I like the book, especially her personal development in Homeopathy. It is very simple and easy to read.

Jan Scholten MD, medical doctor in Homeopathy, researcher, writer, author of *Homoeopathy and the Elements* (*Homeopathie en de Elementen*)

A Little at a Time

Homeopathy for You and Those You Love

A Little at a Time

Homeopathy for You and Those You Love

Mary English

**AYNI
BOOKS**

Winchester, UK
Washington, USA

First published by Ayni Books, 2015
Ayni Books is an imprint of John Hunt Publishing Ltd., Laurel House, Station Approach,
Alresford, Hants, SO24 9JH, UK
office1@jhpbooks.net
www.johnhuntpublishing.com
www.ayni-books.com

For distributor details and how to order please visit the 'Ordering' section on our website.

Text copyright: Mary English 2014

ISBN: 978 1 78535 106 8
Library of Congress Control Number: 2015936386

A CIP catalogue record for this book is available from the British Library.

Design: Lee Nash

Printed and bound by CPI Group (UK) Ltd, Croydon, CR0 4YY, UK

We operate a distinctive and ethical publishing philosophy in all
areas of our business, from our global network of authors to
production and worldwide distribution.

CONTENTS

I would like to dedicate this book to two Homeopaths
Mabel Smith
Janet Snowdon
Thank you for your guidance

Acknowledgements

I would like to thank the thousands of patients I have treated during my 15+ years of private practice. They are truly my teachers.

I would also like to thank my dear friends Usha and Jessica for their Homeopathic support.

This book would never be in your hands without the valuable read-throughs and help from Alam, Han, Kay and Lucy and sound editing from Mollie Barker and all the team at Ayni books including Mary, Maria, Dominic, Stuart, Nick and Catherine.

And lastly I would like to thank Samuel Hahnemann himself, Rest In Peace. Through his infinite wisdom I am a better prescriber.

Preface

Who this book is for:

This book has been written for those people that are interested in Homeopathy. You might already have a good understanding of Homeopathic remedies but might want to learn a bit more about the philosophy of Homeopathy.

You might know nothing about Homeopathy. Then please dive in, this is a good place to start!

If you don't like Homeopathy, or don't want to use it, then I do urge you not only to not read this, but also to not comment or review it anywhere.

Why?

Because it isn't written with you in mind.

I'm not here to convince anyone about Homeopathy's healing powers. I don't want to change anyone's mind. I just want to talk intimately with those that are interested in Homeopathy and who would like to use it in everyday situations and also those who would like to go just that little bit further with their knowledge.

This book does not pretend to replace any health advice you might receive from your doctor or other health professional. What I am hoping to do is help you feel more confident about treating annoying or upsetting but not life-threatening conditions at home.

The biggest cause of unwellness is fear, so I will be showing you plenty of remedies that will help with this.

Introduction

The quantity of action necessary to effect a change in nature is the least possible, and the decisive amount is always the minimum – perhaps an infinitesimal amount.[1]

I would like to tell you a little bit about myself, a little about how Homeopathy found me, and a little about my view of Homeopathy.

Why a little?

Because, as I know, a little can do SO much.

Well, I'm 5 foot!

That's not tall but I've managed to have a career in retailing, have a baby, get divorced, learn to play the Celtic harp, write 14+ Astrology books, make a career change into Homeopathy, and find a lovely new partner and get remarried.

So, what was my introduction to Homeopathy?

I had a baby.

And he had an attack of the croup. I boiled the kettle, rubbed menthol ointment on his chest, nothing worked, he wheezed and wheezed, and I felt powerless and helpless.

A few weeks later I was in the local pharmacy and picked up a leaflet about Homeopathy. It said that Homeopathic remedies were safe for children of all ages and adults too and I read that a remedy called 'Aconite' was good for croup.

I bought a bottle of Aconite 6c and put it in the kitchen cupboard...

And forgot about it.

A few weeks later, my baby boy, now 18 months old, woke me up at about 3am. He was crying and distressed, wheezing and panicky. I then remembered the Aconite I'd bought. I had no idea how to give it to him (he didn't have teeth), but in the heat of the moment I opted to crush one tablet between two spoons and popped the dust onto his tongue...and waited to see what would happen.

In less than 5 minutes, his panicking stopped, his breathing calmed down and then the wheezing stopped too.

WOW! I thought. *This is interesting. Must be something to this Homeopathy.*

That was it.

I was already on my path. It wasn't a linear process, but I started at my local library and read everything they had. The first book was *Lectures on Homeopathic Philosophy* by Kent. Heavy stuff! What was this Pod-ophy-llum he went on about, or Lycopodium?

My interest just grew.

So, here I am after 5 years of training, over 15 years of private practice. Having completed eight provings – and every one I do, I go WOW! Just like I did the first time. They've just had one 6c and all these symptoms came out! How did it do that?

So that's how Homeopathy found me.

A little idea can go a long way. And in the same way, even though we've had a bashing in the press, we're still here. Even though there are some people intent on silencing us and our profession, we still prescribe.

Clients still want to be treated as humans – not as disease labels: the 'eczema patient' or the 'person with M.E.', or the long-name-hard-to-pronounce that we'll find in Black's Medical Dictionary.

We treat people, not diseases: Mrs Black and Mr White and sometimes Ms Grey in-between…

A little at a time.

We don't need banners or flashing lights or white coats to make clients feel better, just friendly smiles and a deep interest in their symptoms.

Our small contributions, our little doses, make big changes to people's lives every day.

When the going gets tough I re-read what Hahnemann said in Aphorism §11, footnote:

The smallest dose of a medicine dynamised in the best manner (where-in, after committed calculation, only so little material can be found that its smallness cannot be thought of or grasped, even by the best mathematical brain) gives out, in the appropriate disease case, more curative energy by far than large doses of the same medicinal substance.[2]

There are big things that can be done with Homeopathy, but we need to do it a little at a time – and this book is to help that process and steer you towards a healthy and successful past, present and future.

A little at a time.

Chapter One

What Is Homeopathy, How Did It Start, Who Uses It?

Before I describe what Homeopathy is, I would like to tell you what it is not.

It's not herbalism, even though a lot of the remedies we use are made from herbs.

It's not always practised by doctors, even though numbers of doctors are trained in it.

It's not expensive, even though paying to see a Homeopathic practitioner might be, depending on what you classify as expensive: about the price of a pair of inexpensive trainers.

It's not like aromatherapy or massage as we don't make physical contact with our clients. They talk to us, and we listen.

It's not, and certainly never will be 'mainstream' medicine, and comes under the banner of an 'alternative' therapy or, to give it its current name, Complementary or Alternative Medicine (CAM).

Let Like Treat Like

Homeopathy is a system of medicine that takes into account the person, not just the disease, and matches like with like. If you were suffering from a high fever, we'd use a remedy that would produce a fever in a healthy person. It's a well-established form of medicine and has been around for 300 years or so.

Short History of Homeopathy

The word Homeopathy comes from the Greek words παρόμοιος or *homoios* meaning 'similar', and ταλαιπωρία or *pathos* meaning 'suffering'.

There are two spellings in use: Homoeopathy and the more

1

modern Homeopathy.

Homeopathy started in the late 1700s when Samuel Hahnemann, a German doctor born in 1755, discovered the first principle of Homeopathy, that Like Cures Like.

After qualifying in medicine Samuel supplemented his income by translating various medical texts. In 1789 when he was 34, Cullen, the author of one of the texts he was working on, stated that the reason Cinchona Bark (*Cortex Peruvianus*) cured malaria was 'because it was bitter'.

In his usual questioning way, Hahnemann didn't agree with this hypothesis, as plenty of other herbs were bitter, but they didn't cure malaria. So he decided to take some doses of Cinchona Bark himself and discovered:

> I became languid and drowsy; then my heart began to palpitate; my pulse became quick and hard; an intolerable anxiety and trembling; prostration in all limbs; pulsation in the head; redness of cheeks; thirst. Briefly, these were all the symptoms usually associated with intermittent fever and they all made their appearance. These symptoms lasted from two to three hours every time and recurred only when I repeated the dose. I discontinued the medicine and I was once more in good health.[1]

The symptoms that the Cinchona Bark produced were exactly the same as the symptoms of malaria. What an amazing discovery! The fact that it produced the same symptoms as malaria itself was the reason it cured malaria. Bingo! This then set Hahnemann on a mission that lasted for the rest of his life.

Minute but Potent

The body is an extremely intelligent thing. It constantly aims for 'homeostasis', a balance in the body so we don't get too hot, or too cold, and we don't fall asleep at our desks (unless we've been out the night before!).

It puts up with lots of abuse from cigarettes, alcohol, lack of sleep and stress; it digests vast amounts of food and sends the by-products exactly where we need them, and it breathes without us having to tell it what to do. Most of the time, for most people, the body works effectively and is always trying to find the best way to keep us alive.

If you've ever watched someone take their last few breaths before death, the struggle the body makes to continue to breathe is mind-boggling. It does all of these things naturally without us having to 'do' anything.

Homeopathy is a safe and effective system of medicine that helps the body's own efforts to heal itself by dosing it with minute 'potentised' quantities of a plant, mineral or animal by-product capable in their undiluted state of creating similar symptoms to those presented by the patient.

Dr Samuel Hahnemann qualified as a medical practitioner in Germany in 1779. During his years as a general physician he grew more and more disillusioned with the profession. He was appalled by the inhumanity and barbarism displayed by the medical practice of his day. Doctors then would use 'treatments' such as bloodletting, using sharp knives or leeches, and massive amounts of laxatives and large doses of medicines, many of which caused serious side-effects. His life's mission was to establish a more humane and natural system of treatment. His pioneering efforts in the face of prejudice and resistance to change brought into being a system of medicine that swept the world and continues to prove effective today.

Having discovered this unusual form of medical treatment, he then devoted the rest of his life to bringing it to as many people as he could. After his first wife died in 1830 he established the first Homeopathic hospital in Leipzig with his friend and assistant Dr Gottfried Lehmann and then spent his final years with his second wife in Paris before he died in July 1843.

Before he died he passed on his experience and ideas to his wife Marie Mélanie d'Hervilly Gohier Hahnemann, to Dr Constantine Hering in the USA, Dr Frederick Quin in the UK, Baron Clemens von Boenninghausen in Germany, and various other doctors and practitioners.

Homeopathy Today

OK, that's Homeopathy's past. What about today? Where is it used and by whom?

In 1999 the BBC conducted a survey to find out what percentage of the UK population uses Complementary and Alternative Medicine (CAM).

Seventeen per cent of the British population use Homeopathic medicines. This survey also found that the average amount of money each CAM user spent on CAM was approximately £14 ($22) per month with a large proportion of users (37%) spending less than £5 ($8) per month.[2]

In the UK there are four Homeopathic hospitals. The one in London is now called The Royal London Hospital for Integrated Medicine, when it was originally called The Royal London Homeopathic Hospital, but to keep the baying hounds at bay, the name was wisely changed.

We still have one in Bristol: The Bristol Homeopathic Hospital, which is near to where I live in Bath and I have referred a number of my patients to their tender, loving care.

There is also one in Glasgow: The Glasgow Homeopathic Hospital, and there is a small one in Liverpool. Just how long they will survive is anyone's guess.

Legally there is no restriction to you having Homeopathic treatment on the National Health Service (NHS). Long may that continue.

The Legal Status of Homeopathy and Homeopathic Practitioners

Homeopathy in Europe

Homeopathy is tolerated in all European countries. Its practice by medical doctors is tolerated in all countries. Practice by professional Homeopaths is also tolerated in a majority of European countries. Only in a small minority of countries, which by law restrict the practice of all medicine to medical doctors, are professional Homeopaths legally unable to practise. Neither the European Commission nor the European Parliament have produced any position statement on who may or may not practise Homeopathy. The delivery of health care services is considered to be a concern of each member state rather than one of the European Union.[3]

Homeopathy in the USA

In the USA there are, as in the UK, medically trained and non-medically trained Homeopaths. Certain states allow it to be practised provided the applicant has also trained in either medicine or osteopathy or veterinary medicine. Thirteen states license naturopathic physicians, and Homeopathy is included within their scope of practice. This exists in the states of Washington, Oregon, California, Idaho, Utah, Arizona, Montana, Kansas, Minnesota, Vermont, New Hampshire, Connecticut, Maine, and in Washington DC.[4]

There are no laws about self-prescribing as the remedies are licensed Homeopathic remedies and are recognised and regulated by the Food and Drug Administration and are manufactured by pharmaceutical companies under strict guidelines.[5]

Well, It's All Just Placebo, Isn't It?

Actually, Homeopathy isn't 'just' placebo.

Here is the official statement from two separate meta-analyses of Homeopathic clinical research trials in 1992 and 1997 which both concluded that

> There is sufficient evidence to suggest that the effects of homeopathic treatment cannot be explained by calling them mere placebo effect but that more research of greater quality needs to be carried out before final proof can be established.[6]

Placebo is the Latin term for 'to please' and implies that a physician is not prescribing a true medicine, but a dummy pill, to keep the patient quiet and happy. But placebos have been proven to be more effective in numerous trials if the prescribing physician is sympathetic and understanding. You know what it's like. You see your doctor and he or she is grumpy and rushes you out of the door. The prescription he/she makes will be ineffective if you have built up an internal resistance to their 'expertise'. Then you visit the locum a few weeks later, and he or she carefully listens to your symptoms; they're sympathetic, caring and understanding about your troubles and you faithfully follow their guidance to the letter.

Which physician will assist your recovery more effectively? Grumpy GP (general practitioner) or Sympathetic Locum?

But Homeopathy isn't 'just' placebo. Remedies can be prescribed to farm animals, babies, plants, domestic pets, racehorses, the unconscious...and they still work!

Research

The European Network for Homeopathy Researchers (ENHR) was established in 2004 with support from the European Council for Classical Homeopathy (ECCH). The ENHR consists of 66 individuals from 15 different countries involved in or with a special interest in Homeopathy research.[7]

Homeopathy and Herbalism

Now, quite a lot of people get confused with what is Homeopathy and what is Herbalism. Homeopathic remedies can be made from anything and are sourced from the animal, vegetable or mineral kingdom, with the majority of Homeopathic remedies made from flowers or herbs. The difference between a Herbal medicine and a Homeopathic one is the Herbal will be made *directly* from the flower or herb, while the Homeopathic will have been diluted and energetically altered. We still use the same sources of plants and flowers but the Homeopathically prepared remedy will have had extra processing to remove side-effects or dangerous poisoning possibilities as some of the flowers and plants we use can kill in their raw state. Remedies like Aconite and Belladonna, which are lethal if ingested, were used by Hahnemann and are still used today, and people are living happy lives from having used them.

Who Uses Homeopathy?

All sorts of people use Homeopathy.

From my case files here is a random sample of the types of people that want to use this natural, gentle treatment. People like you.

Jackie is 45 and has been depressed since her boyfriend left her 3 years ago. Her marriage split in 2001 so she could be with her boyfriend. His leaving has devastated her more than her marriage break-up. Her presenting complaints are: depression, headaches, bad digestion and lack of energy. She has no interest in the physical world.

Rialdo is 32 years old and has come about his stress levels. He is the manager of a sports retailer and is feeling out of control in his work situation.

He is presenting with chest pains and a feeling of tightness in his chest, which he is finding scary and he is very worried. This started 3 to 4 weeks ago and he is feeling more and more tired.

He says he has 'let his guard down'.

Rialdo has stopped training. He runs, enters marathons and is very fit. He enjoys physical experiences, mountain climbing, and camping. Very much an outdoor type. His ambition is to live in a cottage by the sea. He talks at length about how he prefers the sea to mountains. He dislikes lots of people, preferring to be in the company of his wife. Due to the nature of his job, he is in constant contact with lots of people and he is having trouble delegating to others and trusting his team to carry out his wishes. At work he is a perfectionist, wanting to run the best shop in town. He gets on well with his parents and is very close to his dad. His brother recently became engaged and this has caused some family friction. His only fear is of losing his wife.

Georgina is 37 years old. She had an ectopic pregnancy 2 years ago, a termination 5 years ago and a stillbirth last year. She works full time as an administrator for a large government organisation. She has recently given birth to a beautiful baby girl. Since then she has had repeated water/urinary infections, which are making her life miserable.

Lucy is 14 and has had eczema since she was 18 months old. She has it all over her body: ankles, arms, hands, neck, face, in her hair and on her ears and very dry skin on her face. She says it is annoying her and she hates it. She comes from an 'allergic' family: her father had eczema and her older sister has a nut allergy. The pregnancy and birth were fine and she was breastfed. At 1 year old she became allergic to eggs and her lips swelled up. At 4 years old she began to have sleep problems. At 7 years her dog died and her eczema got much worse. She had asthma and was admitted to hospital.

She has had a range of conventional medicines to alleviate her symptoms including Benovate, Ventolin, Diprobase and ultra-violet treatment. She has also tried acupuncture and Chinese medicine. She doesn't like her parents arguing and hates being teased by her dad. She's into horse riding and likes to be outside and active. She's happy when her friends and family are happy.

Claire is 19 years old and studying for a degree at the local university. She has an older sister and two stepbrothers. She has terrible premenstrual tension (PMT) and an irregular menstrual cycle. She grinds her teeth and has to wear a mouth guard at night. She has come about her skin, which makes her feel 'absolute rubbish'. She never drinks alcohol, but she drinks 2 litres of coke or bottled fizzy lemonade a day. She was prescribed a systemic anti-fungal treatment for her skin, but this has made her feel worse. Her stomach is bloated and she feels hungry all the time.

All of these people came to see me for help with their symptoms. They all recovered and are now leading happy, 'normal' lives.

Homeopathy helped.

The major difference between Homeopathic treatment and conventional medicine, or 'Allopathy' as Hahnemann called it, is that we want to understand fully the *person* with the condition or complaint. We don't treat all cases of eczema the same way, as one person might be itchy all the time, and another might only be itchy at night.

We'd select a remedy that has in its profile picture the key symptom 'itchy-all-the-time' for the first patient and 'itchy-in-bed/at-night' for the second.

And how do we know how each of these different remedies will work in different ways?

Because ALL Homeopathic remedies are trialled out on healthy human volunteers before they're used in medical practice and a detailed record is kept of the ways the volunteers reacted to the remedy, which, if we remember that Homeopathic principle, demonstrates what Hahnemann discovered after eating the Cinchona Bark, that Like Cures Like.

It's not only the man in the street who uses Homeopathy; rich and famous people, including the British royal family, do too and when you think about that, it makes you wonder: If Homeopathy was rubbish, why would people pay good money to buy remedies or visit practitioners if the system of treatment didn't work or was ineffective?

Making Sick People Well

So, let's put to one side the idea that Homeopathy is ineffective or useless and go forward with the correct notion that it's an excellent way to regain your health, has no side-effects, is cheap, doesn't hurt the planet, people are not exploited to make the remedies, and all practitioners are motivated by one true desire, the same one that motivated Hahnemann: to make sick people well.

Chapter Two

Main Principles and the Philosophy of Homeopathy

To understand Homeopathy and how and why it works we need to explore a bit about the conventional ideas of sickness.

The World Health Organization defines health as 'a state of complete physical, mental and social well-being and not merely the absence of disease or infirmity.'[1] In that very short and modest statement, there are a lot of grey areas, disagreements and differences.

What you might define as 'being healthy' might be completely different from your friends' or neighbours' ideas of healthy. But until we define what health is, we can't really start talking about sickness or disease.

A good dictionary definition of health is 'a state of being well in body or mind'.[2]

The UK Government department of health doesn't have a definition of health and neither does the USA department of health, which I think is a bit sad. If we don't define health, how can we talk about sickness? They have plenty of information on disease and disease 'prevention' but no definition of what health is.

Some Homeopaths' Definitions of Health

So what do Homeopaths talk about when they define health?

Under the heading 'The Life Force in Health and Disease' Hahnemann, the founder of Homeopathy, has this to say about health:

In the healthy human state, the spirit-like life force (autocracy) that enlivens the material organism as dynamis,

11

governs without restriction and keeps all parts of the organism in admirable, harmonious, vital operation, as regards both feelings and functions, as that our indwelling, rational spirit can freely avail itself of this living, healthy instrument for the higher purposes of our existence.[3]

(*Autocracy:* Supreme, uncontrolled, unlimited authority or right of governing in a single person.

Dynamis: Life force, the force/power/energy which enlivens the material organism.)

What I like about Samuel's definition is that health isn't just about the body, it's about having a connection to 'higher purposes'. So, in a state of health, we're not just being healthy; we can also touch the divine. He must be one of very few physicians to write and talk about not just the physical body but the spiritual.

A modern Homeopath called Vinton McCabe in his book, *Homeopathy, Healing and You*, says health is freedom:

> I am reminded that modern homeopaths often define the word health simply as 'freedom.' The transformation possible allows us to be truly free, not only of physical ailments but also of their causes – anger, fear, guilt, family violence, loneliness, and the like. This is transformation. This is true freedom.[4]

I am in total agreement with this view. Having symptoms and being ill adds to our burden. Being well is being free from pain and anxiety and stress.

Miranda Castro in her wonderful *Mother and Baby: Pregnancy, Birth and Your Baby's First Years* has this to say about health:

> Health is more than simply the absence of disease. I believe it is a sense of well-being, of feeling good, of being in balance, that is hard to dislodge. It is, above all, the ability to withstand stress.[5]

Homeostasis

One thing Homeopaths certainly understand is the body's innate ability to maintain homeostasis. This is when the cells in the body maintain an internal equilibrium by adjusting their physiological processes. This is a dynamic and ever-changing situation kept within narrow limits involving the body's temperature, pH, glucose levels, oxygen and carbon dioxide levels, blood pressure, water and electrolyte concentrations.

When you think about it, considering what actually happens to keep us alive and what our cells and all our bodily functions have to do to keep us breathing, it's amazing we don't malfunction more often! If you really want to be amazed, watch any programme about the moment of conception. That's an amazing feat too…we just don't think about these things often enough. Maybe if we did we'd be more grateful for the health we have and the life we've been given.

Health Problems

Most people don't think about their health, until they get a health problem, which is a shame.

Then there are other people who obsess about their health. They watch every little scrap of food they eat and worry about everything they come into contact with.

A healthier view of health is to not go to extremes, and that applies to Homeopathy as well. If your life is hanging on a thread, don't hesitate to call for an ambulance, but while you're waiting, have some Arnica or Aconite.

I sometimes hear Homeopaths and clients worry that they have to take a course of antibiotics. They worry they'll get even more ill. Let's be realistic here. One course of antibiotics once in a while isn't going to do any harm, but having them every month might. It all depends on your own immunity and your body's ability to excrete the excess drugs from your system.

Hahnemann was against unnecessary and life-threatening

treatments. So taking a drug that might cause you more harm than good is not in my humble opinion a good health choice.

Research Your Drugs!

The other thing to do is to find out about what you're taking. Don't just take your doctor's word for it. Research and look up the drug you're on. The Internet is ablaze with health information. One of the most Googled questions is 'What are the side-effects of XYZ drug?'

So what are the side-effects of your medication? Do you know? How many deaths have been caused because of the drug you're on?

This bit of information from the Medicines and Healthcare Products Regulatory Agency might be useful for you to think about when using prescription drugs:

> Adverse drug reactions are frequently serious enough to result in admission to hospital...Studies performed in an attempt to quantify this have shown adverse drug reactions account for 1 in 16 hospital admissions, and for 4% of hospital bed capacity.
>
> A.D.R.s themselves are also thought to occur in 10–20% of hospital in-patients, and one study found that over 2% of patients admitted with an adverse drug reaction died, approximately 0.15% of all patients admitted.
>
> It is clear that adverse drug reactions adversely affect patients' quality of life...
>
> Adverse drug reactions may also mimic disease, resulting in unnecessary investigations and delays in treatment.[6]

Goodness me! How scary is this statement: *Adverse drug reactions adversely affect patients' quality of life.*

Yes! They certainly do, especially for the 2% of patients that DIED because of the drug/s they were on!

Remember: drugs are made for diseases. Homeopathic remedies are made for people...

The Whole of You

Something that confuses people new to Homeopathy is how a remedy can help more than one health complaint. This is something that puzzled me when I first looked into Homeopathy.

There are websites and books and leaflets that tell you that a certain remedy called Aconite can help with croup, sore throat, swollen tonsils, colic, watery diarrhoea in children, vomiting, high temperature...and fear.

How can one remedy do all that?

In the Western health model, we're led to believe that one product can only do one thing at one time. Don't believe this. It's an out-and-out lie. One product will do lots of things and not all of them are to your benefit!

For instance there are painkillers that are 'only' for headaches and have names like 'Hedex', implying that it will help pains in the head, or 'Propain' that again has the word 'pain' in it, implying it will help sort out pain relief.

Affects, Effects and Bodily Changes

In reality, no drug does just one thing with one area of the body. There are affects and effects, more commonly called side-effects.

Drugs can and will affect the digestive system, the brain, skin, blood, bones, lungs and thinking ability. Every drug you buy or are prescribed will have a sheet in the box telling what the side-effects are. Have you ever read this? I suggest you do and familiarise yourself with the possibility that the drug you are on might be causing you some extra unwanted symptoms.

All of You

Homeopaths already know that ANY substance you ingest will affect ALL of you. It will affect all your bodily systems and your thinking and dreaming, which is why we record all of these symptoms in each proving or drug trial.

So if you have a sore throat and are very anxious about it, as there are more than 50 remedies that would help with the sore throat, we have to find one that has 'fear' in it as well…and also the way the fear is expressed.

Do you want to lie down or move around? Are you quiet or noisy while you're ill?

In the remedy Aconite, the provers were restless, didn't want to be touched and had a great 'sinking of strength'.

Their heads felt full, heavy, pulsating, hot, bursting and burning as if 'the brain were moved by boiling water'.

Their whole bodies were affected from the top of their heads to their feet, with numbness and tingling in their hands and feet, with unsteady knees and a 'sensation as if drops of water trickled down the thigh'.

If we were to sum up the total experience of these Aconite provers we'd use the keywords: mental anxiety, worry and fear.

As Hahnemann said:

Whenever Aconite is chosen homoeopathically, you must, above all, observe the moral symptoms, and be careful that it closely resembles them; the anguish of mind and body; the restlessness; the disquiet not to be allayed.[7]

The Way That You Express It

Another main distinction in Homeopathy is the way that people suffer.

Conventional medicine only covers a person's psyche when they're attending for mental health treatment. Homeopaths do it every day with every case they see.

It's not *what* you've got that we need to treat but the *way* that you express it.

When the provings are conducted, we want to know in what

way are you different from when you started?

- Are your habits the same?
- Are your thoughts the same?
- What person have you become?

It's a well-known fact that people's personalities change when they become ill.

Suffering from a Cold

Three people could be suffering from a cold.

One will want to keep warm and might put on extra clothes and be sitting by the radiator and feeling really chilly. They're worse in the evening, refusing to do things, obstinate; even thinking about, let alone doing, anything physical makes them feel worse.

One might be feeling really hot, throwing off the covers at night because they have such a high temperature and wanting the window open. They're cross, grumpy, furious, biting and striking their loved ones while hallucinating and seeing monsters.

And one might be very fretful and extremely anxious, pacing the room, walking into the kitchen and checking in the fridge one minute, walking into the living room and changing channels on the TV the next. They can't settle and even when they do sit down, they're jiggling their legs or tapping the furniture.

All of them have runny noses, a slight cough, maybe a headache too.

If we just prescribe Aconite for all of them, only the person who is fretful will get better…then comes the cry 'Oh, Homeopathy doesn't work!'

But if we prescribe Calc Carb for the chilly first person and Belladonna for the second, we're making true Homeopathic prescriptions.

We're treating like…with like.

The main difficulty with conventional medicine is that doctors categorise people based ONLY on their diagnosis. And if they don't have a diagnosis, they can't even have any treatment.

Think about the last time a friend or relative went into hospital.

Test Results

There they are, lying on a trolley or in bed on a ward. Unless they've had really obvious symptoms, no-one will tell you what's wrong until lots of 'tests' have been done, lots of blood has been taken and lots of forms have been filled out.

It might be hours or even days before an official diagnosis has been pronounced, while all the time your friend or relative is still suffering with what they came in with. But now they're even more anxious as no-one knows or is telling them what the problem is.

All the heart patients are on the heart ward. All the stroke patients are on the stroke ward. The ones with no obvious symptoms are put on 'observation wards' so the staff can observe how they are over time, in the hope that some 'obvious' disease will reveal itself.

But look at all those patients on the ward your relative is on: do they look or sound the same as your relative?

I expect not…but hospitals are trying to fit them all into the same *disease* model.

When I was diagnosed with diabetes, the ward I was on had an enormous age range of patients. One night the woman in the bed next to me started to become really unwell. She was fighting for breath, making lots of noise, gasping and crying as she felt so bad, and there were no nurses to help as a patient on the next ward was dying.

I spent the night holding her hand and trying to comfort her. In the morning she was told they hadn't expected her to last the night, which is why they had left her, but somehow she pulled through.

She didn't have a diagnosis, they didn't know what was wrong with her, she was elderly and had no family and they just popped her into a bed to keep an eye on her, which didn't happen the night I was there. She was obviously incredibly unwell but because it was late at night, there were no doctors around to 'make a diagnosis' so the nurses were just providing a sort of wait-and-see mentality and as they hadn't expected her to last the night, hadn't arranged a treatment plan.

Without a diagnosis, conventional medicine can't 'do' anything with your symptoms.

Homeopathy doesn't need a diagnosis; it just needs to know all about your suffering, and treatment starts straight away.

Heroic Medicine

I am completely against heroic medicine. Heroic medicine is where a health practitioner does everything and anything to 'help' the unwell person, including treatments that are worse than the original disease.

Surgeon and author Sherwin B Nuland, who taught the history of medicine at Yale, in his book *How We Die* said:

…treatment decisions are sometimes made near to the end of life that propel a dying person willy-nilly into a series of worsening miseries from which there is no extraction – surgery of questionable benefit and high complication rate, chemotherapy with severe side effects and uncertain response, and prolonged periods of intensive care beyond the point of futility. Better to know what dying is like, and better to make choices that are most likely to avert the worst of it…There is another element, too, that these days often conspires to isolate the mortally ill. I can think of no better word for it than futility. Pursuing treatment against great odds may seem like a heroic act to some, but too commonly it is a form of unwilling disservice to patients.[8]

Homeopathy doesn't use this type of energy. It's gentle, calm, natural and uses the smallest amount of remedy possible to help you recover.

Minimum Dose

One thing Hahnemann was at pains to point out was that any treatment a person was given should be the least amount possible to aid their recovery. We don't need heroics to help people recover. It looks good on the telly, lots of medical staff applying electrodes, or administering life-saving equipment to 'ward off' impending death...but in reality, if people were helped a little earlier in their illnesses, there would be less need for heroic, expensive interventions.

Hahnemann, after years of experimentation, discovered that a minimal amount of remedy was needed to gently push the ill person's own life-affirming recovery into action. He'd seen the effects that large doses of poisonous medicines had produced, that bloodletting weakened a person, not helped them.

We don't just need people banging on our chests to recover from heart attacks; we need sensible diets, exercise, reduced stress, and a sense of meaning to our lives...and a little push in the right direction when we start to flag.

It's a bit like flogging a dead horse, or beating up someone who has fallen into a coma. Pushing the river won't make it flow faster, but those same techniques are used every day in conventional medicine. It's as if they're going to FORCE our bodies to recover their health.

Some of the 'treatments' we still use today for cancer patients are nothing short of barbaric and they're all delivered with the idea that cancer needs to be 'fought' and tumours need to be 'battled' as if our bodies are war zones, not intelligent entities.

It's time to stop and take a good long analysis of where our health has gone astray and gently coax it back to wellness.

No-one likes to be forced to 'do' things, and neither do our bodies.

We don't need 50 doses of aspirin for our headache, while running around, staying up late, stressing every time the phone beeps and drinking litres of coke, all of which just makes it worse, when having one dose, a good night's sleep, taking things easier and slowing down a little will do just as well.

We need the minimum amount of intervention possible, and that's the secret to Homeopathy: finding that minimum needed for our own needs.

Hahnemann found that diluting his remedies had a *better* effect than their material doses, but he not only diluted the remedies, he energised them using a technique called potentisation, which I'll discuss later on. Suffice to say here, that less is more.

The Vital Force

Hahnemann didn't just treat his patients. He also wrote a number of books recording his experiences, his theories and his ideas. His first was called *The Organon of the Medical Art*, which Homeopaths shorten to *The Organon* and which is Greek for a series of logical or scientific rules.

In a letter he wrote to his friend Boenninghausen, he said: 'I am at work on the sixth edition of the "Organon", to which I devote several hours on Sundays and Thursdays, all the other time being required for treatment of patients who come to my rooms.'[9]

In it he talked about something he called The Vital Force, or as it was written in German:

Geistartige – spirit-like
Dynamischen – dynamic
Lebenskraft – life force
Lebensprincip – vital principle

These qualities are what living, breathing human beings have and ones that we mustn't forget when we're thinking about treating and helping live human beings.

We're not just lumps of flesh!

Hahnemann was very against the idea of humans just being material entities. He reasoned that there was a spiritual aspect to us. That there was 'something' that motivated us and kept us alive.

I'm sure you've heard many stories about people losing the 'will' to live. Well, that's the Vital Force. Other cultures call it *Prana, Qi* or *Chi*.

There is quite a lot of philosophy in Homeopathy, which I actually really enjoy as it means I'm not just treating people's colds and flus, I'm also considering deeper meaning to their lives.

Samuel made an important point about the Vital Force: 'When a person falls ill, it is initially only this spirit-like, autonomic life force…that is mistuned through the dynamic influence of a morbific agent inimical to life.'[10]

What he meant was in disease *before* the person gets sick, something affects their dynamic self, *then* they get sick. This has been researched and proven in people thinking happy or sad thoughts before being given a flu jab. The people who thought happy thoughts built a stronger resistance to illness than the ones who thought about the sad things that had happened to them.[11]

You'll have experienced this yourself, I'm sure, if you witness someone throwing up.

You're far more likely to want to vomit too, if you see someone else vomiting. There is no exchange of body fluids, no virus to catch, no material reason for it. Just watch someone vomiting and you're likely to vomit too. Even thinking about it can cause it to happen!

This is your Vital Force at work. Your inner alive-ness, your human-ness. It won't happen to your desk or your dining table, but only to you as a human.

Susceptibility

Another consideration we have in Homeopathy is susceptibility. You could have four people all exposed to someone else who is suffering from a cold at work:

- Person One has just been given a pay rise.
- Person Two's dog has just died.
- Person Three is thinking about their up-and-coming wedding.
- Person Four is in a hurry to get their workload for the day finished.

Of these four scenarios, which person do you think is more likely to catch the cold?

Yes! Person Two is most susceptible to coming down with that cold at work.

When we treat someone Homeopathically, we do a thing called 'take their case'. This involves either lengthy questioning in a consultation, or asking the patient to complete a health questionnaire that lists their family health history, their previous ailments, their likes and dislikes, things that affect them, things that make them feel better or worse. Lots of info!

If, say, there is a family history of cancer or heart problems, then they're more likely to either be suffering from that themselves, or need treatment to reduce their sensitivity and susceptibility to these illnesses.

Chapter Three

Homeopathic Provings

Provings are the pillars upon which homeopathic practice stands. Without accurate provings all prescribing indications are bound to be vague guesses at best, and pure fiction at worst. There is no other way to predict the effect of any given substance as a remedy with any degree of accuracy, and the use of signature, toxicology or fancy ideas cannot approximate the precise knowledge gained by a thorough proving.[1]

I have included a whole chapter on provings for one reason only. I know exactly what I'm talking about as I have now conducted eight provings and I'm planning on doing a few more before I retire!

As I mentioned in Chapter One, Samuel accidentally conducted his first 'proving' by ingesting some Cinchona Bark and seeing what happened. The symptoms he produced were exactly the same symptoms that people with malaria produce, so now we know why and how Cinchona Bark helps malaria: *because it has the same effect on the human body.* Like cures like.

This is what we do now before a remedy gets released and I must make a big distinction between a proving and a clinical trial.

Clinical trials of medicines didn't happen until *after* Samuel and his Homeopathic friends started trialling out their remedies before prescribing them. Remember, Samuel was motivated by a strong desire to *not* poison or make worse his patient's state of health. So, the only way to find out the effects that a remedy would produce was to experiment and give them to healthy volunteers.

First of all he used his family, then later on his friends, then as time progressed, he used other Homeopaths and volunteers. He knew that the *only* way to discover a substance's inherent healing qualities for humans was to give a sample of that substance to the volunteer, which is what he did with his first, accidental experiment, then get them to record everything that happened to them after they took a dose.

This still happens today.

The Experiencer

Most good Homeopathic colleges include a proving in the final year of training. This gives trainee Homeopaths a personal insight into the workings of a remedy and puts them into the place of being not the observer but the experiencer.

If you've never taken part in a proving, it's a bit difficult to explain, a bit like me telling you about a new play at the theatre or a new film that's showing. I can tell you and you can hear all about the plot and the characters, but you won't *feel* the emotion or the feelings I felt while experiencing the play or film, and it's those bits that make or break a good production.

When a 'prover' undertakes a proving, they succumb to all the energies of the product and become 'at one' with it. It can be a life-changing experience.

A good, thorough proving will produce numerous symptoms, and will also seep into the minds of the provers, so eventually, they're not sure what's the remedy's effects and what are their own desires.

I would love for more people to experience a proving; then they'll truly understand the weird and wonderful energies that remedies can have.

Samuel originally proved over 50 remedies, quite a task, as he devoted time to developing two a year.[2]

A clinical trial nowadays consists of a number of sick people, all with the same complaint, being given a drug and reporting back if their condition got worse, or better, or stayed the same. As they are *already* unwell, the poor volunteers are just guinea pigs. Some won't even be given the new 'wonder drug', as they are part of the trial called the placebo group.

Volunteers can be paid between £1,000 and £3,500 (about $1,500 and $5,250) for their 'inconvenience'.[3] Most are students at university.

Homeopathic provings are conducted by Homeopaths. I suppose you've got to have a bit of a questioning mind to want to conduct one, as they are time-consuming, brain-frazzling and amazing experiences.

No-one is paid. Not the provers, who are generally friends of the master prover, or students at Homeopathic colleges, not the master prover, nor the pharmacy. There is no money involved, as in reality the only people who will benefit financially from the provings will be the pharmacies, as they have to make and produce the remedies later and some remedies, like drugs, go in and out of fashion.

Some pharmacies potentise the proving remedies for free, so that the Homeopathic community and the general public can benefit from the results.

Win, win.

Unlike conventional medical trials, a Homeopathic proving is aiming to find the healing properties of the substance via a healthy human. I repeat. Human. Not a monkey, or a dog or a rabbit or a fish.

Human.

I sometimes wonder what the rationale is to test a drug on a monkey, when a monkey can't tell you how he/she felt. In a proving, we know everything that the provers felt, in minute detail, because they record all this information in their journals.

My First Proving

My first experience of a proving was at college when we proved Caribou Moss or Reindeer Lichen.[4] The remedy brought up issues of a deep sense of insecurity and procrastination, so could be used to help clients with these issues.

I then conducted my own provings as I found the whole experience so fascinating. The first that I conducted, as opposed to volunteered for, was made from the energies of a thunderstorm and I called it 'Tempesta'.

Then I went on holiday to Wales with my son and found the wreck of the ship *Helvetia*, so I used a small sample of wood from the hull of the boat and sent it to the pharmacy and they made it into a remedy.

My next proving was made from a small sample of loose stone from Stanton Drew Stone Circle in Somerset. Then a sample from Old Wardour Castle in Wiltshire. Aquae Sulis (Bath Spa Water) was conducted alongside volunteers from New Jersey in the USA who also used the same sample of Bath Spa Water.

A sample of rock from the Great Wall of China was given to me by a lecturer in science, and a small sample of sand from Karnak Temple, Egypt was also given to me by a friend who went on holiday there; both were made into remedies and proved.

In 2014 I conducted another proving, this time from a small loose stone from St Michael's Mount in Cornwall.

How a Homeopathic Proving Works

Stage 1

Substance is obtained with permission from owners or organisations and plans made to return substance to source if needed.

Proving substance is sent to Homeopathic pharmacy and made into remedy.

The only person at the pharmacy who knows what the remedy substance is will be the person who actually makes it; sometimes they don't know either.

Numbered remedy bottles are sent to master prover and allocated to each prover.

One will be placebo.

No-one will know which one is placebo, only pharmacist.

Supervisors and volunteers (provers) also don't know what substance is.

Stage 2

Gather together a number of people, mostly about ten.

Appoint supervisors to each volunteer.

Ask provers to commence keeping a journal *before* the proving starts.

Supervisors interview each prover and record their state of health 'before'.

Food likes, weather preference, feelings, current situation, best time of day, previous illnesses, previous medical history, current medication, energy levels, hates, likes, dreams are all recorded. It's a lengthy, detailed process.

Supervisors continue to keep in contact with provers during the proving and phone or meet with them regularly to have them 'feed back' how they are feeling.

Stage 3

Substance is posted or given to each prover.

They are given a time and a date to take first dose of substance.

Proving commences.

Provers write in journals everything that happens to them over the proving weeks.

Supervisors are on call to help provers understand their feelings and ensure they are supported throughout the proving.

Most of the provers won't know the other provers, so they don't exchange ideas or compare notes. This is a solitary process of working with whatever feelings or symptoms are produced during the proving weeks.

Stage 4: Entering the dragon's den

Dreams are recorded, feelings noted, symptoms written down, weather conditions noted, family upsetments, arguments, emotions, etc.

From my experience, after 3 weeks, generally, provers have reached a place of being 'inside' the feeling of the remedy. Now they don't know what is the remedy and what is 'self'.

More questioning happens:

- 'Why me?'
- 'Why this?'
- 'Why now?'

This is a very self-reflective process and demands a lot of the provers. It might not be an enjoyable process and the supervisors are there to support the provers on their 'journey'.

The remedy begins to 'take shape'. Supervisors meet with master prover and discuss 'what is coming up' for the supervisors and the provers.

Proving finishes, provers complete their journals, and post/give them to master prover or supervisor.

Stage 5: Conclusion

Provers and supervisors are told what the remedy was/is.

Supervisors and master prover collate notes.

Provers' journals are copied onto computer and symptoms compared to the 'before' picture of the provers.

Editing, collating, symptom differentiating, discussion, symptoms weighting all take place.

Proving is 'written up' and published for peer review/debate.

Remedy is available at the pharmacy.

Symptoms are then converted into Repertory language. This is the most time-consuming aspect of a proving as the words the provers used have to be converted into succinct, short keywords

– such as: 'Head, pain, worse from heat' – and submitted to editors of the Repertory (book of symptoms).

Keep in mind that the symptoms a remedy can *produce*, in a healthy volunteer, are then an indicator of what it may *cure* in someone suffering from that symptom.

For instance: If you never suffer from headaches and during a proving you develop a hammering migraine, then we know that the remedy has an affinity with headaches.

Provings Today

There are now over 2,000 Homeopathic remedies that have all gone through a similar rigorous process. Some provings only involve a few people. Some have larger amounts of volunteers. I have conducted eight provings to date. They are time-consuming, frustrating, amazing and wonderful experiences and they also need devotion and focus. As I mentioned previously, most colleges now expect third-year students to take part in a proving so they can experience first-hand what it actually feels like to sample a new substance and have it do strange, weird and wonderful things to your body and your mind. This is a collective encounter and knowing that your whole college-year is going through the same feelings as yourself is in some ways more comforting than doing it with people you don't know. In the provings I've conducted, most of the provers don't know each other, but they still manage to produce a 'collective' experience.

Provings can vary considerably in their format and while one proving might be classified as analytical and logical, another might be considered more poetic or creative. I aim for the more creative side of provings because what fascinates me is how there is always one prover who 'speaks' the remedy. They touch in completely with its source, its function, its expression.

The Homeopathic Proving of Aquae Sulis, the Roman Bath Spa Water

The proving commenced on Monday 23rd January 2007. The provers were asked to take the remedy at 9am. Before the proving the supervisors and I 'took the cases' of all the provers so we could get a 'before' picture of the provers' state of health.

The following prover recorded these images after allowing the energies of the remedy to 'take her over' during a meditation just after taking one dose of the remedy. She succumbed to the feelings rather than fought them off with her logical brain.

Prover 9

Day 1

9am Took remedy

9.20am – Meditate – Image of green, tall grass as if I am inside a swamp – breeze blowing the grass above my head. As if I am very small – looking up to this grass and the sky beyond. My Guide took me up and we looked down on tall grass stretching out below us, some bulrushes in there as well. Water – small streams running through.

Now set me down in a deep dark forest – makes me think of rainforest. Very wet, I'm still small, some branches, things seem huge. I could be frightened but I feel secure at the moment. It's warm and damp. This forest, the grass has been here forever, since the planet began.

Stepped into a swampy hole, sucked down. Mouth, ears, eyes filled with swamp. Hands above my head, travelling very fast down a channel of light, feet first.

Deep into the earth, into its core.

Hit rock with a bump. I'm me, but more elemental than who I was, more the essence of me, part of a shaft of light. (Feel tired, heavy – during the meditation.)

Rock is cold, dark like jet, jagged, glistens in the light. Rocky landscape, no sky but light enough for me to see.

Textures important – smooth rock, sharp, jagged, rough, not easy to walk so I sit in one place. No sound, sulphur smell – volcanic? I slip into a crevasse and become part of the rock – shaky, shard, brittle, easily broken up…

Stepping back from meditation now.

9.53am

She relates how she feels after taking the remedy: she is 'sucked down' to the source of where the Bath Spa Water comes from and even notes a smell of sulphur.

The Roman Bath Spa Water smells of sulphur as it contains 1015mg per litre of Sulphate.

Bath Spa water rises at 46° Celsius, the temperature of a hot bath, and contains 43 minerals. The water comes out of the ground at a point where a geological fault (the Pennyquick fault) fractures impermeable strata above the water-bearing rocks, allowing it to rise up from great depth.[5]

This proving ran alongside a proving of the same substance in New Jersey in the USA.

Each prover was given a number between 1 and 12 and this was the only way to identify them afterwards.

Confidentiality was paramount. Things can 'come up' during a proving that volunteers don't want to share. Talking it through with the supervisor, verbalising it, can ensure that only relevant symptoms are published. Keeping a journal can be tedious. Having to write everything you do and feel for weeks on end can seem wearisome, but the more the provers can record, the more we will understand the healing potential of a new substance.

We don't tell the provers what the substance is until after the proving finishes. This is to ensure we don't influence their mental state and make them 'imagine' symptoms. As they have no idea what the substance is, they can just assume that everything they feel is because of the remedy. However, humans are complex beings and during a proving will justify a symptom that has arisen, maybe by saying: 'I feel tired because I stayed up late', forgetting that they've had a new remedy. This is where the supervisors help the provers process their feelings and their symptoms.

This prover kept writing that she wasn't feeling different and nothing was happening:

Prover 10
Day 1
Lots of trouble with the house and a flooded garage – lots of phone calls – I can think of a better way to spend an evening but it did not really affect my mood.

So, even though she *thinks* nothing is happening, as her mood wasn't affected, she's taken a remedy made from water and her garage floods!

This one had a realisation about Homeopathy. He's not a Homeopath, he's a lecturer in science at a further education college:

Prover 11
Day 9
Dreams – still a lot, and detailed – holiday near beach: sudden solar eclipse (unpredicted) – yet I wasn't 'fazed' by this.
Day 15
I'd like to learn more about 'the memory of water' and how Homeopathy might work. But analysis is not the answer!

Before a proving starts we ask the provers about their best time of day, their likes and dislikes, weather, food, sleep and most importantly their dreams.

Dreams from an Aquae Sulis Prover

Prover 9

Day 4

This is based on my concern for a great niece. The dream is set in her house and in the sea. There is contamination in the sea. The great niece collects water in a plastic container and continues to fiddle with it in the house – I didn't recognise her but her mum was there. The great niece develops sores on her arms and she is taken to hospital with smallpox. Her mother is told to clean the house, wash everything. I can't keep awake so occupy a room to sleep. In the early hours, the doctor and other people bring their car with the niece into the entrance hall and have to wait as I have to clean the room I am in – very dusty, messy. In the midst of this, my father goes out, stays out all night and returns to sleep in the early hours.

Day 10

In charge of a school having to organise a day of events. Events happen, everything goes smoothly, I have nothing to do. I give a speech which no-one can hardly hear, but those who do think it's good. A happy contented dream! Needed to find a toilet in the dream.

Day 24

Very mixed with images and people from the day before, plus unknown people and family. The main feeling was getting ready for the wrong thing, in the wrong clothes which kept unravelling and no-one seemed to be able to help, basically not being ready. I needed to wash my hair and in the dream someone gave me a shampoo which made my hair fall out – public place like a swimming pool.

Naufragium Helvetia (Shipwreck)

It's amazing how things change physically for a prover as the proving progresses.

For instance, in the Homeopathic proving of Naufragium Helvetia (Shipwreck) prover number 7 recorded:

Prover 7
Tues 30th Oct: I woke in the night for a wee.
Thurs 31st Oct: I woke up in the night for a wee.
Fri 1st Nov: I woke up in the night for a wee.
Sat 2nd Nov: Took fifth and final pill before bed last night. I woke up in the night for a wee.

After he'd finished the pills this didn't happen again.

Ruina Castellum (Old Wardour Castle)

In the Homeopathic proving of Ruina Castellum (Old Wardour Castle) prover number 2 recorded:

Prover 2
Day 5
I didn't want to eat much when I got home. I seem to have lost my appetite lately. I also don't want to drink coffee. I can't seem to finish a whole cup. I want to eat light foods like salads or vegetables. We have hardly any food in the house because I haven't been bothered to buy any.

In this proving, part of the sample was taken from the dining hall of the castle, where the residents held enormous banquets and feasts.

This is why we talk to provers before the proving starts, so we can establish 'who they are', because as the proving goes on, they can become more influenced by the remedy.

Antidote

On Sunday 12th February 2007 the Aquae Sulis proving finished. We asked the provers to take an antidote of Sulphur 1m before bed. They didn't *have* to take it as some provers have liked remedies so much that they don't want to change things. If they experienced this, then they skipped the antidote, but for those who wanted to go back to the 'way they were', they took the antidote, then recorded their last feelings before bed and on Monday 13th February 2007 posted their completed journals to us.

The remedy was sourced from a sample of water from the Roman Baths and potentised to 30c and 200c at Helios Pharmacy in Tunbridge Wells; the full proving can be read on my website: www.maryenglish.com

The results of these provings now mean I have Stanton Drew Stones to help with extreme fatigue, Shipwreck to help loss of creativity and feeling 'stuck in your life', Aquae Sulis for people wanting to get pregnant, Old Waldour Castle for people trying to 'make a home a castle' or who are homeless or having homing issues, Karnak Temple sand for issues to do with feeling 'sick to death' or mourning someone who has died, Great Wall of China for people feeling persecuted, and St Michael's Mount for people wanting to touch their spiritual life-purpose.

Chapter Four

What Sort of Things
Can You Treat at Home?

This book does not pretend to replace any health advice you might receive from your doctor or other health professional. What I am hoping to do is help you feel more confident about treating annoying or upsetting but not life-threatening conditions at home.

The biggest cause of unwellness is fear, so I will be showing you plenty of remedies that will help with this.

You know what it's like. You find a lump or a bump or something in or on your body that you hadn't noticed before and your mind immediately flips into overdrive and, before you know it, you've self-diagnosed yourself with some cancerous or life-limiting condition.

It's a scary place to be.

When you finally make it to the doctor, with your life-limiting condition you're convinced you've got and he/she says it's 'only' a case of XYZ, you hardly feel relieved because it still hurts or keeps you awake.

Then the inevitable happens.

The Eternal Search

You start searching the Internet. Long hours are spent by people searching the Internet for their symptoms.

Go to any search page and put in 'Pain in…' and you'll see the options come up: Side, Arm, Shoulder, Breast.

Now put in 'Extreme pain in…' and you'll get: Lower back, Stomach, Shoulder, Foot.

Those search terms only come up because so many *other* people have been searching for that information too.

Even if you find a website that describes your symptoms adequately, you then start searching for 'Treatment for...XYZ' and even more options will come up.

And do you feel any better 'knowing' all this information? Do you feel relaxed now that you 'know' that you've got XYZ?

I expect you'll be like most people and feel even *more* anxious or concerned.

When I'm helping a client with their health issues, I often send them information on charities that help. Most charities are there to help the person suffering from XYZ and aren't there to make a profit, unlike the hundreds of advertisers that place their adverts near or next to the searches you've made for medical advice on Google.

And not every one of those advertisers is altruistic in their motives. They're there to make a profit and, in some cases, big profits.

I agree with Dr DM Gibson who says in his *First Aid Homoeopathy in Accidents and Ailments*: 'Long experience has proved the value of certain remedies in relation to all manner of accidents for the purpose of countering shock, allaying pain, arresting bleeding, preventing infection and speeding convalescence.'[1]

I'm not saying that you're going to become a brain surgeon overnight with a Homeopathic first-aid kit, but you are going to feel less helpless and more empowered.

The sort of things you can safely treat at home are those things that your GP is unlikely to want to see you in the surgery with. Anyone that has a runny nose, coughs, sneezes, or has spots or a fever will not be too welcome. These are things you can safely treat provided they haven't been going on for too long...and too long is more than a week.

Self-Help

Self-help is a wonderful resource and one I use myself a lot. I'd much rather read some nice friendly introduction to something and learn it in my own time, at my own pace, than have someone pontificate to me face to face and not understand what I actually need help with.

I am writing this book from that place.

I would like you to imagine I am there, on and by your side, giving you advice but not forcing you to do anything against your will. I might make suggestions, I might recommend, but always you have the choice to either accept or reject my advice.

What I do have to share with you are my own personal experiences *as a client* and the personal experiences *of my clients* and my experience of *treating my clients*.

Those are three different viewpoints:

1. Me – the client
2. You – the client
3. Me – the practitioner

I am writing this book to help you help yourself in whatever way you'd like, using Homeopathy as a resource.

Losing Confidence

We seem to have lost the confidence to treat certain things at home.

I suppose what makes it worse is the bewildering amount of products and info you can be subjected to on the Internet, or even in a chemist shop.

I worked in a chemist when I was in my late teens. I was trained in serving customers but had to work out myself what products were suitable for various ailments.

We had drawers behind the counter with products labelled from A to Z and in there were the things we couldn't put on the shelves. If a customer asked for something with a P on the packet, it meant it could only be sold if the pharmacist 'oversaw' the transaction.

In reality, we only had to hold up the packet and he/she would either nod or shake their head and we'd give it to the customer to buy (or not).

We hardly asked the customer any questions. We didn't ask how long the problem had been going on, what made it better or worse, or what other symptoms they had. When I think today of what we *didn't* ask, compared to what a well-trained assistant might ask today or a Homeopath asks, it's rather scary.

Gaining Responsibility for Your Own Health

The best way to feel empowered about your own health is to remember that your body is a very intelligent piece of kit. People have had reasonably healthy bodies since the human race began and they've either looked after them and had good health, or they've pushed their bodies to the limits and suffered from long-term health complaints, or worse, died from their lifestyle choices.

You know as well as I do that smoking is the biggest cause of ill health. How can it not be? If I stood you in front of a bonfire on a really hot day and forced you to breathe in the smoke, I'm sure you would feel sick, dizzy and short of breath, but people every day put cigarettes in their mouths...and breathe in the smoke.

And I did that too!

Don't ask me why I did. I don't have any idea! All I know is cigarettes were available, I could buy them from the corner shop, they didn't cost too much money and before I knew it I was 'a smoker'.

According to the World Health Organization:

Tobacco use is a major cause of many of the world's top killer diseases – including cardiovascular disease, chronic obstructive lung disease and lung cancer. In total, tobacco use is responsible for the death of about 1 in 10 adults worldwide. Smoking is often the hidden cause of the disease recorded as responsible for death.[2]

I eventually stopped smoking when I read a book called *The Only Way to Stop Smoking Permanently* by Allen Carr.[3] I expect he saved my life. I know he saved his own. I used to drink coffee. Almost every day. Cappuccinos galore. But I got terrible verbal diarrhoea, asthma and anxiety and eventually I stopped.

Hahnemann, I later discovered, was so anti-coffee that he wrote a short book called *Treatise on the Effects of Coffee* in 1803.[4] He classed coffee as a medicinal substance, or what we would call an over-the-counter-drug now: 'It is especially dangerous to make dietetic and frequent use of purely medicinal substances endowed with great strength.'

If I can stop drinking it, you can too.

Then I discovered that my eczema would improve if I stopped eating dairy products like cheese and milk. So I stopped eating them as well.

I now do my best to look after my body. I work with it, not against it.

You can for quite a few years punish your body but you can't do it for too long; something will give. So there is no good 'taking a remedy' for indigestion if the easier solution is to eat less to start with.

Be responsible for your own health. You'll feel better. Your life will be easier. You'll spend less money on over-the-counter medications and you'll sleep better. Even if you have a long-term medical condition you have been born with, you can still be healthy in your mind and body. Doesn't that sound better?

Home Complaints

The sort of things you can treat at home are the sort of things you're probably already treating such as headaches, tiredness, sleeplessness, backache, skin rashes, small cuts, grazes or bruises, coughs, colds, and various pains here and there.

One thing I would like you to do before you start using Homeopathy is to promise me you won't try 'converting' other people to its use.

Lots of clients of mine, when they've had successful treatment with Homeopathy, send all their friends and relatives to see me, promising them that I will help whatever condition they have. I will certainly help, no doubt about it, but Homeopathy works best when people discover for themselves, through their own investigation, that this very strange but simple form of medicine is very effective, cheap, and even, may I say it, fun!

So keep this information to yourself. Keep it safe in your mind and use it for a while to gain an understanding of how it and our bodies work; then, if you really must, tell your friends, but only if they *ask* how you managed to overcome your skin condition or health concern.

Accidents and Injuries at Home

According to The Royal Society for the Prevention of Accidents (RoSPA)[5] the majority of accidents in the home occur in the lounge/study/living/dining/play area parts of the home with the kitchen being the second most likely location. Forty-six per cent of those accidents were some sort of a fall. In 20% of accidents in the home the person was 'struck' by something moving or static.

The types of injuries people suffered were 'open wound', 'bruise/contusion', 'other soft tissue injury' and 'joint, tendon and bone injury'.

The areas of the body most affected were the:

- Arm or upper limbs – 36%
- Leg or lower limbs – 32%
- Head/face – 23%

Of those, 45% were treated at a hospital Accident & Emergency department and needed no further treatment, 21% were referred on to an outpatient clinic, and 12% were referred to their GP. The remaining were admitted as an inpatient, referred to another hospital or referred to a specialist hospital. Interestingly, fewer than 4% didn't *wait* to be treated!

The biggest type of injury was 'open wound' with 'soft tissue injury' coming in second place.

So, what does this tell us?

We're more likely to have an injury in the home than we are out shopping, or being at work, and since this book is written to help those 'at home', I really strongly suggest you get yourself a first-aid kit, lots of bandages and gauze or large non-stick dressings, learn some first aid and keep your remedies handy; you never know when you're going to need them!

Chapter Five

What Not to Treat at Home

After using Homeopathic remedies for a while, you can get quite confident. This is good. What isn't good is when you think you can safely treat something but completely overstep your actual ability.

There are plenty of books and websites that will give you step-by-step home-help suggestions for very serious conditions, but to attempt to treat them successfully at home is, in my opinion, playing with fire.

I met a man in a pub when I was in my third year of training. I used to run a folk club in this pub and was in there to organise the next month's event. This gent had had a bit too much to drink and was in a rather maudlin state and, as usually happens if I stand anywhere for too long, decided to tell me his complete medical history. I have no idea why he decided to pick on me; I wasn't even talking to him!

Terrible Eczema

Anyway, he told me he suffered with terrible eczema. He was top to toe in itchy, red outbreaks. He said a friend had suggested he get some Homeopathic Sulphur, so he bought some tablets from the local health-food shop and commenced taking the tablets.

He took them daily for a month. He said after a few weeks, his skin cleared up! Completely! He was *so* amazed! Eureka!

His skin was smooth, the itch had gone and he felt all was well in his world...except he carried on taking the tablets.

Now, he said, his eczema was worse than ever and the itch had come back and the tablets were 'not working any more'. He had no idea why they had 'stopped working'.

I took a deep breath and explained that they *had* worked, but what was happening now was he was 'proving' the medicine. He needed to stop taking the tablets.

'Stop?' he asked. 'Why?'

As I was in a rush, I didn't know him, he wasn't a client of mine and in his inebriated state he was unlikely to remember anything I told him, I just repeated he needed to *stop* taking the tablets. If he had been to see a Homeopath, she/he would have noted the return of symptoms and stopped prescribing the remedy, but because he was 'home-treating' himself, he didn't have that objective ability or even the experience of how remedies work to make things better.

Becoming Competent

When you're dealing with a health condition, knowledge of the workings of remedies, the way the body copes with stimulus, and a million other things is necessary before you can become competent in 'helping' yourself or others.

I remember when I first noticed Homeopathic remedy descriptions, I thought: *How can Aconite help terror, anxiety, restlessness, fear of death, suppressed periods, high fever, hot skin AND croup? How can one medicine do so many things?*

I'd read in Homeopathic leaflets that the remedy Pulsatilla was recommended for acne, menstrual problems, arthritic aches and pains, and would wonder: *How the hell can one remedy help all those conditions?*

It didn't make sense.

The Way It Is Expressed

After I learned more about Homeopathy I realised that it wasn't *what* the specific condition was that each remedy would help, it was the *way* that it expressed itself that was important.

Equally, when you self-treat or use remedies at home, you can experiment with different remedies until you hit on one that works, but to be a better prescriber, choose one that helps in a *specific* way.

Also, don't carry on taking remedies for months on end, or you'll end up like the man I met in the pub, having all your symptoms return, and be 'proving' the remedy.

So how do you know when to safely treat at home and when to call an ambulance, visit your doctor or call a professional Homeopath?

Homeopaths talk a lot about conditions that are 'chronic' or 'acute'. What is the difference?

Acute Complaints

An acute condition comes on suddenly and the patient either recovers or dies. Most home-treatable conditions are acute...and hopefully the patient doesn't die!

You don't usually die of a cough or a cold, but a cough or a cold could lead to bronchitis or pleurisy and that's where home treatment stops.

Here are a few illnesses that you *must* seek medical attention for:

Meningitis

The symptoms are a severe and rapidly developing feeling of unwellness, including feverishness, listlessness, a severe headache, vomiting, sometimes neck pain, sometimes a dislike of bright lights, feeling very sleepy, vacant and/or confused, sometimes fits.[1]

Septicaemia

Vomiting, fever, limb, joint or muscle pain, fast breathing, rash (anywhere on the body), cold hands and/or feet, very sleepy, vacant, confused, delirious, fast breathing and/or breathless and/or pale skin.

Stroke

Remember FAST:

- Face: Ask the person to smile. Does one side of the face droop?
- Arms: Ask the person to raise both arms. Does one arm drift downward?
- Speech: Ask the person to repeat a simple phrase. Is their speech slurred or strange?
- Time: If you observe any of these signs, call for help immediately.[2]

Heart attack

The symptoms of a heart attack vary from one person to another. They may feel tightness, heaviness or pain in their chest. This may spread to their arms, neck, jaw, back or stomach. For some people, the pain or tightness is severe, while other people just feel uncomfortable.

As well as having chest pain or discomfort they may become sweaty, feel light-headed or dizzy, or become short of breath. They may also feel nauseous or vomit.[3]

Severe asthma attack

The main symptoms are:

- Reliever isn't helping or symptoms are lasting over 4 hours
- Symptoms are getting worse: cough, breathlessness, wheeze or tight chest
- Too breathless or it's difficult to speak, eat or sleep
- Breathing may get faster and it feels like they can't get their breath in properly
- Children may complain of a tummy ache.[4]

Life-threatening symptoms for babies (0–3 months)

The following symptoms and signs are suggestive of potentially life-threatening physical conditions in a baby.

A major change in the baby's behaviour, for example:

- less active than usual
- less responsive than usual
- more irritable than usual
- breathing faster than usual or grunting when breathing
- feeding less than usual
- nappies much less wet than usual
- has blue lips
- is floppy
- has a fit
- has a rash that does not fade when pressed with a glass
- vomits green fluid
- has blood in their stools
- has a bulging or very depressed fontanelle
- has a temperature higher than 38 °C
- with the exception of hands and feet, feels cold when dressed appropriately for the environment temperature
- within the first 24 hours after the birth:
  - has not passed urine
  - has not passed faeces (meconium)
  - develops a yellow skin colour (jaundice).

Other life-threatening symptoms

Tenderness and pain in the back of the lower leg, chest pain, shortness of breath, or coughing up blood.

These are symptoms of a potentially dangerous blood clot in the leg, especially if they come after sitting for a long time, such as on an aeroplane or during a long car trip. These signs can also surface in someone bedridden after surgery.

Chronic Complaints

A chronic condition is one that comes on slowly, and the patient never truly recovers. They're still alive but their overall health and well-being has severely reduced. They might overcompensate for their condition. Go up stairs less, go out less, be home more, or watch what they eat or do. Chronic conditions are what most professional Homeopaths see in private practice, but these are not conditions you can treat yourself forever because:

a) You're too near to the disease or condition to accurately assess it

and

b) How are you going to know how much remedy to take or when?

However, you can start using a home-treatment plan for a chronic condition if you keep in mind that at some point in the future, you will almost certainly need professional help.

There is one major rule: If on taking a remedy there are NO signs of improvement in the next hour, then seek help.

Seek Help Symptoms

The symptoms you need to be aware of that you can't treat at home are anything that is completely unusual to the person. Such as any pain that isn't relieved by taking remedies, especially if accompanied by abnormal behaviour, an abnormal discharge, high fever, difficulty breathing, unconsciousness, swelling, blueness of the skin, diarrhoea, severe itching, extreme tenderness on movement or touch, or vomiting.[5]

You can always take some Aconite yourself if your partner or child is seriously ill, just so you can keep a clear mind while you wait for help.

Chapter Six

The Whole Person, What Is It, and How Do I Treat It?

Conventional medicine can be viewed as reductionist. It categorises patients into disease-labels, and keeps them there. You cease to be a 'person' and instead you become the asthmatic, the alcoholic, the diabetic or the eczema sufferer.

With this style of approach it's hardly surprising that the general public can become a little disillusioned with Allopathy, the term Hahnemann used to describe conventional medicine.

It is true that medicine has advanced far beyond our original expectations. We can look at babies in the womb, stitch missing limbs back on, clone human cells, but with all this advancement we seem to have lost the reasons for having a Health System.

Allopathy views disease as something to be eradicated. The disease is something that comes from outside the person and a cure is the removal of the symptoms. Again, this is a rather limited viewpoint because it ceases to address the major factor: the person suffering from the disease.

Homeopathy views symptoms as the body's way of expressing an internal malady.

A cry for help!

It also has a much different attitude to disease. This is viewed more as a *process* that the person goes through, not what they are. Almost as if disease is a journey.

In Homeopathy, cure is a restoration of health. A return to the healthiest state that the person is capable of. The balancing of the person's energy, making them more able to deal with their own symptoms and have their own body deal with and remove them. When the 'internal malady' has been resolved, health can be restored.

An example of the Allopathic approach would be as follows.

It All Started with Hay Fever

Louise has been suffering from hay fever since she was 2. It started when her younger brother was born. She was treated with antihistamine, which removed the itchy eyes and runny nose but caused her to feel drowsy. She spent most of her summers indoors.

By the time she reached junior school she had developed eczema. Her skin was very red and itchy and she scratched most of the time. This was treated with a well-known cortisone cream.

At puberty she was still suffering from hay fever and still using antihistamine. At 15 she started to smoke and developed asthma and became increasingly allergic to cats, dogs and feathers. She was now treated with inhalers. One for attacks, one as a preventer.

By the time she's in her early twenties she is even more allergic and has become emotionally unstable. She complained to her doctor that she was depressed and anxious. This got worse and her lifestyle became erratic until eventually she was diagnosed as bipolar. She was prescribed anti-anxiety medication and tranquillisers. She is sedated to calm her down.

One year later she develops diabetes and becomes insulin-dependent.

In Homeopathy we understand that Louise's original internal malaise was never dealt with properly. There was a family history of hay fever: her grandmother suffered from it and her father had a severe bout of eczema when he was working abroad in the tropics. This was so severe that he needed hospitalisation.

Miasmatically, Louise was susceptible to being allergic. The birth of her brother was her first experience of jealousy and she dealt with it by developing hay fever. The watery eyes and runny nose are similar to the symptoms of grief and weeping.

More Vital Organs Affected

Unfortunately the medical treatment Louise received pushed the illness back further into her psyche and she became progressively worse. The illness began to affect more vital organs, in this case her lungs. Her symptoms were displayed on a physical level and were being treated on that level even though they originated on the emotional level with the birth of her brother.

Louise's Vital Force was still strong enough to display more symptoms, and even though her Vital Force was being suppressed she now expressed symptoms on the emotional level by becoming excitable. This is a much more serious matter because the illness had now reached her inner being.

She 'became' emotional because her inner being was struggling to be heard.

When these symptoms arose, again they were mistreated and she became mentally unstable. Then the drugs she received for the bipolar destroyed a vitally important organ, her pancreas, and she developed diabetes, a difficult condition to reverse.

All of this was caused because of the original treatment for her hay fever.

Can you understand the gradual reduction of her health and the increase in her unwellness?

Is hay fever such a life-threatening condition that it needs such strong drugs to control it?

At no time was Louise's treatment individualised by listening to her family inheritance and understanding her childhood jealousy. How different this case could have been if she had been treated Homeopathically at the beginning! A sobering thought.

However, recent Homeopathic treatment brought a lessening of her emotional angst and a complete recovery from her allergies. She now owns a cat!

Her eczema and hay fever and asthma have all cleared. Also, Homeopathic treatment has achieved an overall lessening of insulin requirements and a stone (14 lb) in weight reduction.

Is this cure?

It sure as hell looks more favourable than a life of allergy and upsetment!

It also goes to prove that treating mental, emotional *and* physical symptoms brings about a better state of health. In every case we treat, the patient just wants to be heard. Be it by what they say, or what their symptoms say. The language of Homeopathy is to treat the person, not the disease, and to recognise what the symptoms are saying.

Identifying the disease does not explain its origins or help its cure.

There are major differences between the conventional and Homeopathic approach.

Conventional medicine seems better suited to acute, life-threatening conditions where intervention is the only option, e.g. major car accidents, fire injuries, drownings, war injuries, broken bones and impact injuries.

Homeopathy, however, has the ability to lessen the effects of trauma or acute illnesses – but I know I would prefer a surgeon to stitch me up if I got squished by a car!

Both forms of medicine have their place. Homeopathy isn't the answer to Life, The Universe and Everything, but it does address with more empathy the suffering that humans have to cope with. Conventional medicine, with its lack of under-standing the whole person, does us a disservice. Until we under-stand the person behind the disease we cannot hope to cure...and cure should be our highest ideal.

The Whole Person

So, when a Homeopath talks about the whole person, what they mean is they take into account not only the person's constitution but also their life circumstances.

We weigh up what is most important.

We ask the important question: What needs to be cured?

If you were to fall down the stairs, giving a remedy for tooth pain will not address the current problem. However, administering a few doses of Arnica while you ring for the ambulance would help the most.

When we make a judgement on a remedy to give someone, we must take into account the type of person needing the remedy.

If you have a headache and you're normally a fast-talking, fast-working, suspicious type of person, your headache would be more suited to the remedy Lachesis. While your husband, who also has a headache and has just had two bottles of wine at lunchtime, and three strong Americanos since breakfast, might need the remedy Nux Vomica.

Both of these remedies will cure a stonking headache, but using different remedies for the different *personality type* will bring a better result.

Symptoms can manifest in any part of the body and they can move from one place to another, but most of the time, you'll be expressing those symptoms *in the same way*. It's that 'you', that 'same-ness', that we're treating in Homeopathy. The part of you that's individual to you and about you. Homeopathy truly is an individual therapy, which is its major strength.

So, when we choose a remedy, it has to have something about the 'you' of you in it.

The Totality of Symptoms

In addition to treating the whole person, Homeopaths also aim for treating the totality of symptoms: all the symptoms and signs of a disease.

It's no good prescribing or using a remedy such as Belladonna for a hot throat and tonsillitis if you *don't* have a high fever, don't *feel* hot or are white as a sheet.

If you're all shivery, cold, and walking from room to room, it doesn't matter so much about the tonsils thing...using Arsenicum would work better.

So how do other Homeopaths describe this totality of a person's symptoms?

Dr RAF Jack in his *Homeopathy in General Practice* gives a lovely example of a person complaining of nausea. If we were to look up remedies that have nausea as a proving symptom, we'd find hundreds of remedies. But if the person

> has a headache, has become extremely irritable and unsociable, is offended at the most harmless word (like a 'bear with a sore head') and is hypersensitive to noise and smells; if he feels unusually chilly, has a sore throat...cannot sleep at night and is worse in the mornings, then Nux Vomica is probably indicated. Here the choice is made by mental and general symptoms rather than by the particular one of nausea.[1]

He then goes on to describe how if this person were to have conventional treatment, he'd be prescribed a medicine for the headache, given lozenges for the sore throat, a tranquilliser for the irritability and a sleeping tablet for the insomnia, and says: 'How much simpler to give one medicine that covers the totality of his symptoms, all of his symptoms, by using Nux vomica.'[1]

Robin Logan in his *The Homoeopathic Treatment of Eczema* describes totality in this way:

> It is my view that the totality has no boundary. Our understanding of the totality is determined only by our ability to perceive it. Thus Hahnemann uses the phrase in Paragraph 12: '...manifestations accessible to our senses...'[2]

Vinton McCabe in his *Homeopathy, Healing and You* says:

> As we begin a homeopathic healing, we look at the symptoms that are troubling and put them in the context of all the other, more benign symptoms that are also being presented. This

complete picture is called the *totality of symptoms*, which represents the patient's true state of being and a road map for the homeopath to follow in the selection of appropriate remedies.[3]

So, treating the whole person means finding a remedy that has in its proving symptoms the essence of the person, and to make an even better prescription, we can treat all of those symptoms, the totality of the person, not just a few bits and bobs here and there.

Then we have complete health.

Chapter Seven

Everyday Diseases and Complaints:
How to Recognise and Treat Them
Homeopathically

To safely treat an illness at home, you first of all need to remember what I mentioned in Chapter Five about what *not* to treat at home.

Don't mess about if someone is in *extreme* pain, as any sort of pain is an indicator of a serious condition.

Also anything that doesn't show *some* sort of improvement in a maximum of 2–4 hours might be more serious and need hospital attention.

Before you home prescribe, think: 'Is this something *my/their* body is capable of healing?'

Most of the time, our bodies will aim for homeostasis, and will do their best to get better.

If we have a virus, we'll produce a nice high fever to burn off the onslaught. If we cut ourselves, our bodies will send extra blood to the area, making it swell and form a scab until new skin grows underneath.

However, in both of these examples things could need expert help. A fever that continues for hours will eventually cause dehydration or brain and/or heart problems. A cut that is more than a few millimetres deep will need plugging with dressings or stitching.

You can safely prescribe for those things you might already have home remedies for, and colds are top of that list.

There is an old saying that colds go in a week if you don't treat them or seven days if you do! I don't know if I completely agree with that, as I've seen colds clear up very nicely in a day or so with the right remedy.

A cold is when there is a runny nose, maybe a slight temperature, maybe a sore throat, a feeling of unwellness and lack of an appetite. As colds are so individual, keep in mind the type of cold that it is, and the type of person suffering from the cold.

The top 12 diseases/complaints you can safely treat at home in alphabetical order are:

Acne
Back pain
Colds
Constipation
Coughs
Dermatitis
Diarrhoea
Headaches
Heartburn
Indigestion
Sprains and strains
Vomiting

To treat these conditions Homeopathically, you need to ask yourself some questions: Where? When? How?

- Where is the complaint located?
- When is it worse or better, or what makes it worse or better?
- How does it make you feel?

A Homeopathic prescription is based on you, the person suffering, not on what the complaint is called.

You can't prescribe too deeply just on 'I've got a cold; what remedy do I need?' We need to ask: 'When did it start, what part of the body is affected, when is it worse or better?'

So, for the common cold, we could ask: 'When did it start?'

If it started after spending a morning in cold air, playing in the park, we might think of using Aconite, also if the symptoms came on suddenly.

If your nose is really runny, with lots of fluid pouring out, we might think of using Nat Mur.

If you're grumpy, like a bear with a sore head, and feeling very cold and shivery, we'd think about using Nux Vomica.

Homeopathic Literature

A lot of Homeopathic literature was written in previous centuries.

The biggest outpouring of books was in the late 1900s by wonderful authors such as Phyllis Speight and Dr Dorothy Shepherd. Most of the books Homeopaths use to learn from today were written in the late 1800s and early 1900s as Hahnemann died in 1843 and James Tyler Kent died in 1916.

Does that matter?

No, I don't think it does as we're still humans living in human bodies, wanting to recover and get better.

If something can stand the test of time, and in Homeopathy's case, hundreds of years, then it must help in some way. However, because some of these books were written so long ago, the language has changed considerably and we find authors writing about 'carriages' instead of cars, or 'fireplaces' instead of radiators, or 'letter writing', which has surely nearly died out with the advent of computers and mobile phones!

Comforting Care

What certainly hasn't changed one iota is when someone is ill they want comforting and care, good care. Remember, Homeopathy isn't mainstream; in the UK it's certainly niche. And we've got more money here for expensive, time-consuming treatments while in places like India it's more widely used than in the West, because it's much cheaper.

When selecting a remedy keep in mind not so much *what* the condition is that you're treating but the *way* it's being expressed.

One thing that beginners find terribly hard to understand is how one remedy can help more than one condition. How mad is that?

The reason for this is because *any* medicine is going to affect more than one area of your body. Conventional medicine divides us into pieces and treats each of those pieces. A pill for your headache, a cream for your skin, an inhaler for your asthma, and so on.

However, the reality is any medicine will affect all of your body.

We are told that drugs have 'side-effects'. They don't. They have 'affects'.

Side-Effects

Here is an official list of 'side-effects' of the 'common' painkiller ibuprofen.

Common side-effects of ibuprofen include:

- nausea (feeling sick)
- vomiting (being sick)
- diarrhoea (passing loose, watery stools)
- indigestion (dyspepsia)
- abdominal (tummy) pain

Less common side-effects include:

- headache
- dizziness
- fluid retention (bloating)
- raised blood pressure
- gastritis (inflammation of the stomach)
- duodenal or gastric ulcers (open sores in the digestive system)

- allergic reactions, such as a rash
- worsening of asthma symptoms by causing bronchospasm (narrowing of airways)

Less common side-effects can also include malaena (black stools) and haematemesis (blood in your vomit). These side-effects can indicate that there is bleeding in your stomach.[1]

As you can see from the list above, the medicine you may be taking for your headache may also affect your digestion, your blood pressure, your skin and your breathing. It can make you dizzy, nauseous and give you diarrhoea and fluid retention. We might have made access to over-the-counter medicines far easier, but at what cost?

In proving the Homeopathic remedies, the Homeopaths discovered that every part of the body produces symptoms. Maybe Homeopathic remedies will affect some parts of the body more than others, but affect the body they will.

To make selection easier I've divided the following list in two ways. You can search for your condition/complaint or you can read the description for each remedy and decide which one fits your experience best. 'Worse' and 'Better' are when the person themselves feels better or worse in certain situations. For instance, a person needing Gelsemium will feel better *in themselves* when they urinate a lot, or a person needing Sulphur will feel worse *in themselves* when standing up. This has nothing to do with their symptoms, just how they feel psychologically.

Top Ten Home Remedies and How They Can Help

Aconite
Full Latin name: Aconitum Napellus
Monkshood; Ranunculaceae
First line of defence for any sudden shock or anxiety-producing situation.

Complaints caused by exposure to cold dry air, or exposure to draughts. For people with a sense of great fear and anxiety of mind. They are afraid to go out. They are restless, anxious, doing everything in great haste; must change position often; everything startles them.

Pains are intolerable, driving them crazy, becoming very restless at night.

Fever: skin dry and hot; the face red, or pale and red alternately; burning thirst for large quantities of cold water; intense nervous restlessness, tossing about in agony. Their complaints become intolerable towards evening and on going to sleep.

Useful for children that are teething, that are fretful, are screaming, with hot dry skin and high fever.

Coughs and croup that is dry, hoarse, suffocating, with loud, rough croaking, and/or whistling on breathing out. Complaints come on after being outside in dry, cold winds or from draughts of air.

Symptoms made:

- Worse – Evening and night, in a warm room; when rising from bed; lying on the affected side.
- Better – In the open air.

Arnica
Full Latin name: Arnica Montana
Leopard's Bane; Compositae
Made from a small, yellow, Swiss mountain herb. Used by sportspeople worldwide, athletes, even skateboarders, this is the top home remedy for all sorts of bashes and bumps that you, members of your family or your children might get. It's available as a cream or lotion but used as an internal remedy can be more effective. Fantastic to use after a long gardening session too. Jolly useful if the person falls over or has an injury and then immedi-

ately stands up and says there's nothing wrong with them, when obviously there is! If you've got jet lag, try a few doses to reduce exhaustion.

Use it when there is any mechanical injury, even if it was received years ago.

There is a sore, lame, bruised feeling all through the body, as if they've been beaten. Where there is traumatic pathology of the muscles. Think of Arnica when someone has concussion or contusions and for the results of shock or injury. They are nervous and cannot bear the pain. Their whole body is oversensitive.

They can have belching and the burps smell foul and putrid, like rotten eggs.

Use it when there is dysentery; with urine retention, with fruitless urging and/or a long interval between stools.

Constipation where the rectum is loaded and faeces will not come away.

Great for soreness of the personal parts after giving birth.

Useful for when there is retention or incontinence of urine after giving birth.

Symptoms made:

- Worse – At rest, when lying down, from wine.
- Better – From contact, motion, moving about.

Belladonna

Deadly Nightshade; Solanaceae

Its common name is Deadly Nightshade, which you might have heard of. The plant is highly poisonous in its natural state but once made into a Homeopathic remedy, it brings comfort and relief for a number of conditions.

When the symptoms are hot, with red skin, a flushed face, glaring eyes and an excited mental state, Belladonna works really well. A great remedy for high temperatures in children or adults. If all the senses are hyper, with delirium and restless sleep, with a dryness of the mouth and throat and an aversion to water, use this remedy. There can also be neuralgic pains that come and go suddenly.

Use when there is a headache, with a red face, throbbing of the brain and the carotid arteries supplying the head. They feel worse from the slightest noise, motion or lying down and are made better from tight bandaging, or wrapping up.

Symptoms made:

- Worse – From touch, motion, noise, draught of air, looking at bright shiny objects, after 3pm, night, after midnight, while drinking, uncovering the head, summer sun, lying down.
- Better – At rest, standing or sitting erect, warm room.

Coffea

Coffee; Rubiaceae

This is one remedy anyone who lives a busy lifestyle should have in his or her Homeopathy first-aid kit. As it's actually made from coffee, it's jolly good when you've overdone the stimulants and need a bit of a detox.

Use it when the person is completely oversensitive with all their senses more heightened: including sight, hearing, smell, taste and touch.

They might have unusual activity of the mind and body with fainting or trembling.

Use Coffea when the ailments come from the bad effects of sudden emotions or pleasurable surprises. They can weep from delight and alternate between laughing and weeping. Their pains are felt intensely, driving them to despair.

When someone is sleepless, in a wide-awake state, finding it impossible to close the eyes, Coffea calms. There is physical excitement through a mental state of extreme happiness.

Headache: from over-mental exertion, thinking, talking; one-sided, as if a nail were driven into the brain, worse in open air.

Toothache: intermittent, jerking, relieved by holding ice-water in the mouth, but returns when water becomes warm.

Watery, painless diarrhoea.

Symptoms made:

- Worse – Noise, touch, odours; cold, windy open air. Mental exertion, excessive emotions (joy). Overeating, alcohol, wine.
- Better – Lying, sleep, warmth. Holding ice in mouth.

Gelsemium
Yellow Jasmine; Loganiaceae
Another flower remedy and great for the flu when all you want to do is lie down and be left alone because everything aches so much.

There is a desire to be quiet, to be left alone. They do not wish to speak or have anyone near them. There is an overpowering aching, tiredness, heaviness, weakness and soreness felt in muscles of the limbs.

Use Gelsemium when there is anticipation of any unusual ordeal, such as preparing to give a speech, in church, theatre, or to meet someone for first time, that is so bad it brings on diarrhoea. Helps calm the nervous dread of appearing in public or for actors suffering stage fright.

There is great anxiety about the present and the future.

There can be vertigo. The headache feels as if there is a sensation of a band around the head.

Chill without thirst.

Symptoms made:

- Worse – Emotions, dread, shocks, ordeals, motion, surprise, thunderstorms, bad news.
- Better – Profuse urination, sweating.

Ignatia

St Ignatius Bean; Loganiaceae

This is one of my most favourite remedies. One I would take to a desert island. It works so effectively for any kind of emotional trauma. When there is a loss of a family member or relative, death of loved one, or at the ending of a relationship.

This remedy has great contradictions, with a roaring in ears that is better from music, piles that are better from walking, and a sore throat that feels better from swallowing!

Use it for people who are mentally and physically exhausted by long-concentrated grief. When the anger, grief or disappointed love has caused a bad effect for the person. They have a desire to be alone but they can be inconstant, impatient, hesitant and quarrelsome.

Remember Ignatia when there is involuntary sighing.

Symptoms made:

- Worse – From tobacco, coffee, brandy, contact, motion, strong odours, mental emotions, grief.
- Better – Warmth, hard pressure, swallowing, walking.

Ipecacuana

Ipecac; Rubiaceae

This is one of the top nausea remedies. The remedy is made from the root of a small, shrubby plant found in most parts of Brazil.

When there is persistent nausea, with profuse saliva, vomiting of white mucus in large quantities without relief and feeling sleepy afterwards, this is the remedy to consider. They might be feeling sick because of the effects of tobacco or during pregnancy. There is a sinking sensation in the stomach that feels like squeezing and griping. There are cutting pains across the abdomen from left to right. When the person is vomiting during pregnancy and in some cases more nausea than vomiting.

Their stool grassy-green, white mucus, fermented, foamy and slimy. They are oversensitive to heat and cold.

Symptoms made:

- Worse – Slightest motion, warmth, damp, overeating, ice cream, pork, veal, mixed or rich food, candy, fruits, raisins, salads, lemon peel, berries, lying down
(Nothing in particular makes this person's symptoms feel better.)

Nat Mur
Common Salt; NaCl
Great remedy and has been in use for hundreds of years. Made from common sea-salt. When you think about how salt is used as a preservative, you will understand how the signature of this remedy matches the patient's desire to hold onto and remember past hurts. Pain is preserved and rarely let go of. It has been said that this is a typical English remedy as the English are so 'stiff upper lip' and averse to expressing their true feelings.

When the person is suffering from a complaint that has been brought about by the ill effects of grief, fright and anger, Nat Mur brings relief. They are depressed, particularly when they are suffering from chronic diseases. Consolation aggravates and makes them feel worse. They want to be alone to cry.

They have throbbing headaches, from sunrise, to sunset, with a pale face, nausea and vomiting. Their headaches are periodical and are from eyestrain and during menstruation. The eyes feel bruised and give out when reading or writing and appear wet from tears.

There is ringing and noises in the ears. Their lips and corners of their mouth are dry, ulcerated and cracked.

They have an unquenchable thirst. They crave salt. There are cutting pains in abdomen. When there is painless and copious diarrhoea alternating with constipation with dry, crumbly stools, think of Nat Mur. They can have irregular menses that are usually profuse. The cough has a bursting pain in head. There can also be a fast beat of the heart.

When there is a pain in the back, they desire firm support to make it better. They can have eczema that is red raw with inflamed skin.

Symptoms made:

- Worse – From noise, music, warm room, lying down, at seashore, from mental exertion, consolation, heat, talking.
- Better – In the open air, cold bathing, going without regular meals, lying on right side, pressure against back and tight clothing.

Nux Vomica
Poison Nut; Loganiacea
Another wonderful remedy well suited to 'modern' life when the person overdoes stimulants, is hurried, angry-with-everyone-and-everything and is very impatient. Great for hangovers or when you've eaten too much, especially highly seasoned or spicy foods.

It is made from the seeds of a medium-sized tree that mostly grows in India. The seeds are highly poisonous in their natural state.

They have an oversensitiveness to external impressions: to noise, to odours, light or music; even the smallest ailments are unbearable. The teeniest comment will set them off. When you've overdone too much coffee, tobacco, alcoholic stimulants, highly spiced or seasoned food, Nux Vomica will settle things down. When you've overeaten or spent long amounts of time being mentally over-exerted (think exams, study or extreme computer work) or you have sedentary habits with no exercise, too much sitting or suffered loss of sleep, this is the remedy to help.

Their pains are tingling, sticking, hard, aching and worse from motion and contact.

When there is constant nausea after eating, in morning, from smoking and a feeling of 'If I could only vomit I would be so much better', then use this remedy.

They have constipation with frequent unsuccessful desire and pass only small quantities of faeces and then have the sensation as if not finished. There is a frequent desire to pass stool that is anxious and ineffectual.

They alternate between constipation and diarrhoea.

When menses are too early, profuse, last too long, or keep on several days longer, are irregular and never at the right time, stopping and starting again, Nux Vomica is fab.

They have backache that makes them sit up or turn over in bed. They can have lumbago.

They absolutely hate the cold or cold air and feel chilly. The least movement is unbearable and they hate being uncovered and must be covered in every stage of fever.

There can be fever, great heat, with the whole body burning hot, the face red and hot, yet the patient cannot move or uncover without being chilly.

Symptoms made:

- Worse – Morning, waking at 4am, mental exertion, after eating or overeating, touch, noise, anger, spices, narcotics, dry weather, in cold air.

- Better – In evening, while at rest, lying down and in damp weather.

Sulphur

Brimstone; Flowers of Sulphur; The Element

This was one of Hahnemann's first remedies and it is a fab all-rounder. Helps when other remedies slow down or cases need cleansing from overdosing.

It is sourced from volcanic activity found near hot springs and volcanic craters in Sicily, the USA and the Italian peninsula. It is then chemically purified and ground into a fine powder so that it is soluble in water and alcohol.

Helps when cases relapse, when carefully selected remedies fail to act, and is often of great use in the beginning of treatment of chronic cases and for finishing acute ones.

We used this a lot when we worked in a drugs and alcohol detox day centre.

People that need Sulphur are very forgetful and find it difficult to think. They are busy all the time. They think rags are beautiful things, so you'll find them keeping things that you might consider should be thrown away! They are averse to business; they loaf around and are too lazy to rouse themselves. They can be irritable, depressed and can get thin and weak, even with a good appetite.

They have a sick headache that recurs periodically. They are oversensitive to odours, even though they may themselves be dirty and unwashed.

Their lips are dry, bright red and burning. They have a complete loss of or excessive appetite. Milk disagrees and upsets their stomach so they can vomit it up. They feel very weak and faint at 11am and must have something to eat.

People that need Sulphur have itching and burning of the anus, piles and a frequent unsuccessful desire to pass stool. Children needing Sulphur will be afraid of the pain when passing a stool. They have morning diarrhoea that is painless, but drives them out of bed. They can have bedwetting because of a sudden desire to urinate.

Their menses is preceded by a headache. Also if the menses suddenly stops, this remedy will help.

They have difficult respiration, so they want the windows open, and there is much rattling of mucus. It feels as if a load is on the chest.

They have trembling of the hands and burning in soles and hands at night.

Sulphur has vivid dreams. They wake frequently and become wide awake suddenly. They can also have catnaps. The slightest noise wakes them up. There can be night sweats. Disgusting sweats that smell of sulphur. When the skin is dry, scaly, unhealthy, itching, burning and worse from scratching, think of Sulphur. They can have pimply eruptions, pustules and hangnails.

Symptoms made:

- Worse – At rest, when standing, warmth of bed, washing, bathing, in morning, 11am, from alcoholic stimulants, periodically.
- Better – In dry, warm weather, lying on right side, from drawing up affected limbs.

Common Home Complaints

Here are the same remedies listed by complaint:

Acne

- Arnica – Itching, burning, eruption of small pimples. Crops of small boils. Deep-seated acne: this is characterised by being symmetrical on the body.
- Belladonna – Acne of the cheeks and nose. Erysipelas:

bacterial infection of the skin. Skin dry and hot.

- Nat Mur – Oily, shiny skin on face. Greasy skin.
- Sulphur – Dry, scaly and unhealthy skin, pimply eruptions, pustules, skin worse from using creams, ointments, and/or washing.

Back pain

- Aconite – Numb, stiff, painful. Crawling and tingling, as if bruised. Bruised pain between scapulae.
- Belladonna – Stiff neck. Pain in nape, as if it would break. Pressure on dorsal region most painful. Lumbago, with pain in hips and thighs.
- Gelsemium – Dull, heavy pain. Dull aching in lumbar and sacral region, passing upward. Pain in muscles of back, hips, and lower extremities, mostly deep-seated. Muscles feel bruised.
- Nux Vomica – Backache in lumbar region. Burning in spine, worse 3–4am. Cervico-brachial neuralgia, worse when touched. Bruised pain below scapulae. Sitting is painful.

Colds

- Aconite – Very runny nose with much sneezing, throbbing in nostrils. Nosebleeds of bright red blood. Mucous membrane dry, nose stopped up, dry or with scanty, watery coryza (snot). Complaints caused by exposure to dry, cold weather, draught of cold air. Fever that has cold sweats and icy coldness of face. Coldness and heat alternate. Chilly if uncovered or touched.
- Belladonna – Coryza with mucus mixed with blood. The throat feels constricted with a desire to swallow but sensation as if a lump was there. High fever but no thirst.
- Gelsemium – Dizziness, drowsiness, dullness and

trembling. Watery discharge from nose that burns. Difficulty swallowing, especially of warm food. Throat feels rough and burning. Fever; wants to be held because he/she shakes so. Muscular soreness, great prostration and violent headache. Nervous chills.

- Nat Mur – Violent, fluent coryza, lasting from 1 to 3 days, then changing into stoppage of nose, making breathing difficult. Discharge thin and watery, like raw white of egg. Violent sneezing coryza. Infallible for stopping a cold commencing with sneezing. Loss of smell and taste. Fever comes with violent thirst. Chill between 9am and 11am.

Constipation

- Ignatia – Itching and stitching up rectum. Stools pass with difficulty. Painful constriction of anus after stool.
- Nat Mur – Constipation, stool dry, crumbling. Burning pains and stitching after stool.
- Nux Vomica – Constipation with frequent ineffectual urging, incomplete and unsatisfactory, feeling as if part remained unexpelled. Passing only small quantities at each attempt. Constriction of rectum. Scanty stool with much urging. Constant uneasiness in rectum.
- Sulphur – Itching and burning of the anus with piles. Frequent, unsuccessful desire to pass stool that is hard and knotty and insufficient. Child afraid on account of pain.

Coughs

- Aconite – Hoarse, dry, croupy, hacking cough, loud laboured breathing. Child grasps at throat every time they cough. Cough worse at night and after midnight. Tingling in chest after coughing.
- Belladonna – Tickling, short, dry cough at night. Barking

cough, whooping cough. Moaning at every breath.

- Gelsemium – Dry cough with sore chest.
- Ignatia – Dry, spasmodic cough in quick successive shocks. Coughing increases desire to cough. Hollow spasmodic cough, worse in the evening, little expectoration, leaving pain in trachea.
- Ipecacuana – Cough incessant and violent with every breath. Chest seems full of phlegm, but does not yield to coughing. Suffocative cough, whooping cough, with nosebleed, and also from the mouth. Rattling cough. Croup.

Dermatitis/Eczema

- Belladonna – Skin is dry and hot. Sensitive, burns scarlet, smooth. Eruption like scarlatina suddenly spreading. Boils. Alternate redness and paleness of the skin.
- Gelsemium – Hot, dry, itching, measles-like eruption. Livid spots.
- Nat Mur – Dry eruptions, especially on margin of hairy scalp and bends of joints. Fever blisters. Urticaria where the skin itches and burns. Eczema that is raw, red and inflamed, worse from eating salt, or being at seashore. Greasy skin.
- Sulphur – Skin itching, burning, worse when scratching and washing. Itching, especially from warmth, in evening, often recurs in springtime, in damp weather.

Diarrhoea

- Aconite – Watery diarrhoea in children. They cry and complain much, are sleepless and restless. Stool is green, like chopped herbs. They can collapse with much anxiety and restlessness.

- Belladonna – Thin, green, dysenteric, in lumps like chalk. Shuddering during stool. Stinging pain in rectum.
- Gelsemium – Diarrhoea from emotional excitement, fright, bad news. Stool painless or involuntary.
- Ignatia – Diarrhoea from fright. Haemorrhage and pain, worse when stool is loose.
- Ipecacuana – Stools pitch-like, green as grass, like frothy molasses, with griping at the navel. Dysenteric and slimy.
- Sulphur – Morning diarrhoea that is painless but drives them out of bed. Burning and pressure in rectum during stool, burning in anus after stool.

Headaches

- Aconite – Burning headache, as if brain were moved by boiling water. Fullness, heavy, pulsating, hot, bursting, burning, undulating sensation. Intercranial pressure.
- Belladonna – Much throbbing and heat. Palpitation reverberating in the head with laboured breathing. Headache from suppressed catarrhal flow. Pain worse from light, noise, sudden movements, lying down and in the afternoon.
- Coffea – Tight pain, worse from noise, smell, narcotics. Seems as if brain were torn to pieces, as if a nail were driven into head.
- Gelsemium – Dull, heavy ache. Bruised sensation. Headache with muscular soreness of neck and shoulders.
- Ignatia – Feels hollow, heavy, worse stooping. Headache as if nail were driven through the side. Congestive headaches following anger or grief, worse, smoking or smelling tobacco.
- Nux Vomica – Oversensitiveness. Scalp sensitive. Congestive headache, associated with haemorrhoids. Headache in the sunshine. Pressing pain on vertex, as if

nail driven in. Frontal headache, with desire to press the head against something.

Heartburn

- Aconite – Tachycardia: fast heartbeat. Problems of the heart with pain in left shoulder. Stitching in chest. Palpitation, with anxiety, fainting and tingling in fingers.
- Nat Mur – Heartburn, with palpitations.

Indigestion/Dyspepsia

- Ignatia – Much flatulence. Cramps in stomach, worse from slightest contact. Averse to ordinary diet, longs for a great variety of indigestible articles. Craving for acidic things.
- Nux Vomica – Ravenous hunger, especially about a day before an attack of dyspepsia. Upper and middle part of the abdomen bloated with a feeling as if a pressure from a stone, several hours after eating. Dyspepsia from drinking strong coffee. Difficult belching of gas.
- Sulphur – Great desire for sweets. Colic after eating.

Sprains and strains

- Arnica – After injuries, falls, blows, contusions. Especially suited to cases when any injury, however remote, seems to have caused the present trouble. After traumatic injuries, overuse of any organ, strains. Sore, lame, bruised feeling.

Vomiting

- Aconite – Vomiting, bilious, mucous and bloody, greenish. Drinks, vomits, and declares they will die. Vomiting, with fear, heat, profuse sweat and increased urination.

- Arnica – Vomiting of blood. Fetid vomiting.
- Belladonna – Nausea and vomiting. Great thirst for cold water. Empty retching. Uncontrollable vomiting.
- Ipecacuana – Persistent nausea and vomiting
- Nux Vomica – Sour taste, and nausea in the morning, after eating. Nausea and vomiting with much retching. Wants to vomit, but cannot.

How to Take a Remedy

Your remedy will be in a glass or plastic bottle. Sometimes they are produced in a 'click pack' where you hold the bottle upside down and click the lid and a tablet pops out into the lid. If you're using this method, just undo the lid and put the tablet into your mouth, chew it slowly, without washing down with water as the tablet will be absorbed through the lining of the cells in your mouth. They don't need to be digested like conventional tablets. If your remedy comes in a normal bottle, just tip the tablet into the lid to avoid handling it too much and then pop into the mouth.

Potency

Homeopathic remedies that are made for the general public, in tablets, come in two different potencies: 6c and 30c. We call these low potencies. Higher ones are available from Homeopathic pharmacies, but they need supervision by a qualified Homeopath.

When you're treating at home, repeat every hour or so until relief. As the remedy kicks in, slow down repetition. This is a completely different way of taking a medicine to conventional medicine.

You're not going to be ingesting the actual flower or mineral, you're going to be swallowing something made from it, but in a highly diluted, energised form. So you have to think about the energy of your symptoms needing to be matched by the energy of the remedy.

The more tablets you take, the more you're inputting an energetic imprint into your body. The more intense the symptoms, the more often you can repeat as the energy of the illness will burn up the remedy.

Like starting a log or coal fire, you'll need a few, quick repeated doses to start, then when the repetitions match the energy of the 'burn' you can reduce as the 'fire' gets ablaze and the person's Vital Force completes the cure. As you start to recover, repeat less frequently until you start to feel better, then STOP.

Quantities

Three tablets are no better than one tablet as you need *doses* of a remedy, not *amounts* of tablets. So repeating every hour for 3 hours is more effective than having three tablets all at once.

Remember: STOP taking the remedy once symptoms get better.

Chapter Eight

Childbirth, Early Parenting

The birth of a child is normally a wonderful happening. I say 'normally' because most people are anticipating and looking forward to the birth of their offspring. However, sometimes pregnancy can be unplanned or even not wanted.

I will cover all options.

What is important is to take your time making a decision about pregnancy. A child is for life and that's a minimum of 18 years! So before you step into the world of mother and fatherhood, be sure you can imagine your child growing up, leaving home, getting a job and possibly getting married or having a partner, and later even having children of their own.

I'm not going to repeat the wonderful works of other authors in this field as I'm not really qualified to write too much about it from my own personal experience.

My pregnancy didn't quite go the way I imagined it. I ended up with an elected caesarian section. And this was before I knew about Homeopathy, so I didn't even have remedies to help me afterwards! Mine was a purely medical matter. I opted for a TENS machine to help with my contractions but since the birth didn't progress in an accepted way, or in accepted timings, I was booked in for surgery at 4pm. My lovely son was born 40 minutes later.

I suppose writing about pregnancy is a little like writing about weddings. There are so many different approaches and options. And also like weddings, it's not the birth that matters, it's afterwards, the marriage, the long-term effects on you and your health and the health of your family.

Unplanned Pregnancy

An unplanned pregnancy can bring a whole host of unwanted emotions. These ladies and gents would benefit considerably by using Ignatia to help their emotions while they give themselves time to make their decisions:

My partner Louisa, who I've been dating since last year, is going to have a baby. Yes, this is unexpected and unplanned, but we are going to come together and do what is best for each other and the child. We think the child is due in April of next year. So there's lots of work for us to do between now and then, including arranging for Louisa to move here to Arkansas. It's all rather overwhelming, really.

I found out I was pregnant 4 days ago with my first baby (7 weeks gone). I am 23 and not with the baby's dad. I don't know what to do. I'm leaning more towards keeping the baby at the moment. However, I have told my parents and they're not being very supportive. They've said they couldn't cope with a baby and how it isn't fair on them. They've said I'll be ruining my life, I won't cope and I'll end up alone with no prospects. They said what have they done wrong as parents in the last 23 years to deserve this. Dad said Mum couldn't cope if I continued with the pregnancy and I said 'Well, that's her problem' and he said 'Well, in that case you deserve to be alone and struggling if that's your attitude.' I just don't know what to do. Everyone else has been supportive so far and my sister has even said I could go and live with her if I do continue the pregnancy. I don't have a lot of money but I do work at the moment in a supermarket. I really want to keep my baby but they keep trying to tell me how awful it will be. But maybe they're right? I don't know.

Unwanted Pregnancy

An unwanted pregnancy delves even further into desperate feelings, which need to be resolved first before sensible decisions can be made. Having some time to make up your mind and having someone unconnected to you to talk to is very important. The Samaritans helpline can help with this. Call 08457 90 90 90 in the UK or 1 (800) 273-TALK in the USA.

Just found out I'm pregnant (not planned) and feel so annoyed with myself for being in this situation. I already have two beautiful children with my husband. I thought I was finished with babies. I'm due to start college in September and my husband has started his own business. There is a long list of why we shouldn't go through with this pregnancy: money, the house would be a bit of a squeeze, the list goes on. I have booked a termination but can't help feeling upset and torn. Me and my husband just can't make this big decision. It makes it harder because I'm reaching 30 so I know I won't be having any more babies and when I look at my two children I feel I'm being selfish even considering termination.

I want to die. I can't handle having a termination. But I have no choice...Life for life.

There is no right or wrong way to deal with pregnancy news. There are better or worse ways of being pregnant or giving birth but, as these examples show, there are many multiples of emotions that surround the whole subject of birth and babies.

On the one side we have 'babies are cute and cuddly' and on the other we have 'babies are monsters that will ruin my life'. The reality lies somewhere in-between.

Let's assume that the pregnancy you have is proceeding well.

Childbirth for Dads

Some dads can feel a little left out while their partner is giving birth. Afterwards there is so much to do, but leading up to the birth, you will feel better when you have something to 'do' too.

Getting a Homeopathic home birth kit to administer (even if you're not having a home birth) will help you have a plan of action if or when your partner loses the ability to speak for herself.

If the only remedies you remember to use are Ignatia, for when she gets upset and weepy, and Arnica for after the birth, you will have found a wonderful way to contribute to the birth of your child.

It can be really helpful to give yourself jobs to be 'in charge of' during labour. This can be a great way to be actively involved in the birth. Look up coping techniques and relaxation techniques – practise them throughout the pregnancy so you are an expert on the day!

Other jobs:

- Find out how to apply counter-pressure on the back
- Acupressure or reflexology points
- Massage
- Different birth positions

If she is using a Homeopathy birth kit, read through the information and be in charge of administering the remedies. Best to buy pills that dissolve easily as she may not have the concentration to chew.

- Create the right atmosphere – get music she loves, anything else that is important to her
- Be in charge of taking pictures or videoing
- Make sure she eats/drinks
- Fill the bath or birthpool and empty it afterwards

- Take the weight off her – find a supported stance

Ensure you both have healthy snacks and drinks for energy, and don't go hungry yourself.

Healing after the Birth

After the birth you can use these Homeopathic remedies to help:

Arnica – Relieves the soreness and bruising and helps with after-pains. It is also helpful for babies who are bruised from a long labour or a forceps delivery.

Bellis Perennis – To help with bruising to deep muscle tissues; use after Arnica if you are still sore after a few days.

Belladonna – Think about heat! Belladonna is a key fever remedy that aids sudden eruptive fevers and inflammatory conditions marked by great redness, heat, throbbing and a thirst for cold water. It is also great for red hot spots from teething, boils, abscesses or tonsillitis. Don't underestimate its throbbing pains, especially the dizzying headaches that will not let you bend over without thinking your head will burst. Sun exposure may contribute to symptoms needing Belladonna, as can light, noise or sudden movement.

Belladonna may be called for in cases of mastitis where your breasts are red-streaked from the centre to the circumference, inflamed, hot, tender, engorged and throbbing with pain. Your milk supply is over-abundant and you are emotionally excited with a high fever with dry, burning heat, red face and dilated pupils. Lying down makes you feel better.

Chamomilla – In the UK this is sometimes called 'Teetha' and is made from the herb chamomile for teething babies. Chamomilla is sensitive, irritable, thirsty, hot and numb. The child wants many things which they then refuse: the classic giving the child a toy, which he/she then throws out of the cot or buggy, then cries to have the toy back. The child can only be quietened when carried about and petted constantly.

Gelsemium – Great for post-natal exhaustion, slow pulse, tired feeling and mental apathy. Lack of muscular co-ordination. Muscular weakness. General prostration. Sensation as if uterus were squeezed.

Kali Phosphoricum – Mental exhaustion after the birth with headache. When there is insomnia, feeling sleepy but too excited to sleep, especially in the first few days after the birth.

Nat Mur – For anaemia, great debility with weakness felt in the morning in bed. Great weakness and weariness of the person and the body. Very oversensitive. Weeps in private.

Phosphorus – Mammary abscess. Infection of the breasts, with a burning, watery, offensive discharge and pus. Use this also if there is a slight amount of blood from the uterus between periods.

Pulsatilla – For post-natal 'blues', especially when the milk comes in. They feel utterly miserable and are bursting into tears at the slightest thing. They weep when talking and feel much better for being comforted. They can be ill-tempered and resentful. They want to be out in the open air and always feel better there. Thirstless and chilly.

Sepia – When there is weariness and misery and a bearing down sensation as if everything would escape through the vulva. They must cross the limbs to prevent everything falling out or press against the vulva. They are worse from doing the washing and the laundry work. Indifferent to those loved best and can lose affection for their partner. They don't want to do anything. Intolerant to anyone in the family. Weeps when telling symptoms.

Silcea – Nipples very sore, ulcerated easily, drawn in. Discharge of blood from vagina every time child is nursed. Hard lumps in breast. Fistulous ulcers of breast. Itching of vulva and vagina, very sensitive.

High Fever in Children

Normally speaking, a fever is a sign that the body is trying to fight off an infection by raising the body's temperature to kill any bugs. In cases of fever in children, more than an hour of a high fever is not only exhausting for a child but also very scary for a parent, so don't try and treat very high fevers.

The average 'normal' temperature is between 36.9 and 37.5 °C (98.4 and 99.5 °F).

If nothing is happening and the temperature isn't coming down, do ring your local doctor for advice.

Tepid Sponging

If there are no other symptoms apart from the high temperature, you can undress the child, lay them on a clean towel on the floor in a warm room, and sponge their face, arms and legs and front of the body with tepid water. Then turn the baby/child over and wet sponge the arms, legs and back and then pat gently dry.

Repeat six times.

Give the baby/child as much to drink as they want, such as water or very diluted apple juice or low/no sugar squash.

If still no improvement, call your GP/hospital.

I also really recommend all parents have first-aid training, as knowing what to do in an emergency not only gives you confidence to deal with something while you wait for help but makes describing or dealing with the problem much easier. Details of training are in Chapter Fifteen.

Alternative Contraception

One thing I would like to suggest if you're not planning on getting pregnant at all or again are the alternatives to the pill, implants, and contraception. There is an alternative and I used it all the time after having my son until I reached menopause because I didn't want to have any more children.

It's called a Persona machine. Here's the website link: www.persona.info/uk/

In the USA it's called Clearblue: www.clearblue.com

I only mention this as I have a number of clients who don't want to be taking chemicals to control their periods and also don't want over 300 shots of that chemical in their body each year. The Persona or Clearblue machine tests your wee and gives you an instant result and, provided you follow the instructions, you will be as safe as you can be in your cycle. NO form of contraceptive is 100% safe, but this little machine can save lots of heartache, and chemical intrusion.

Chapter Nine

Physical Problems
with Suggested Remedies

I have listed the physical conditions by body part, from the head down to the toes.

I've included remedies in this chapter where you don't have to take into account the 'totality' of the person and can just prescribe nice and easily for the condition that you are suffering from. These would be classified as first-aid remedies. They can be used to help make each of these conditions more bearable and might even hurry them along, curtail them or even nip them in the bud.

In Homeopathy, we list the arms, legs, hands etc together in the Repertory and call them the 'extremities'.

The most-used first-aid remedies in my home are Arnica, Aconite and Nux Vomica for bruising, shock and overeating/indulgence!

Keep in mind that any symptoms that don't get better from using these remedies will need professional help. Plus if you've suffered from them for any length of time, then they're not really acute complaints and would come under chronic, which would need someone else to treat effectively. However, you won't harm yourself by using them.

Most high street shops will stock these remedies in the 6c or 30c potency. In the UK you can buy them in health-food shops like Holland and Barrett, in some chemists like Boots, in specialist shops like Neals Yard, or even some supermarkets.

I have listed in Chapter Fourteen more places you can use online.

You can repeat a 6c quite frequently, one tablet every hour if something is really troublesome. A 30c is best taken a few times a day, maybe two or three times: before breakfast, lunch and/or dinner/tea. Take the remedy in a clean mouth (without anything else in your mouth at the time) and just chew it slowly until it's dissolved.

The remedy is absorbed through the lining of the cells in your mouth and does not need to be washed down with water. Try not to swallow the tablets whole; they don't work if you do that!

Stop Taking the Remedy When You Feel Improvement

The trick to Homeopathy is to repeat the remedy until you feel some improvement, and then *stop*.

There is no point in continuing to take a remedy when you can feel it's started to work. Be sensible. Taking remedies all the time will only result in you proving the remedy; see Chapter Three for more information on this.

In Homeopathy we can differentiate a condition by how it started. So say, for instance, you had a headache after spending the last 2 hours dancing (yes, there is a remedy for this!) then you could use the remedy Argentum Nitricum which has in the Materia Medica the following: 'Head – Headache from mental exertion, from dancing'.

So, someone somewhere, while they were proving this remedy, got a headache after going dancing...that's how specific Homeopathic prescribing can be.

Remember: Not all headaches are the same!

Head

- Headache
  From alcohol – Ruta, Nux Vomica
  From eyestrain – Gels, Nat Mur, Ruta
  From sleep loss – Nux Vomica
  From sunlight or heat – Belladonna, Gels, Nux Vomica

Type of pain:

Aching, dull – Aconite, Belladonna, Gels, Ignatia, Nux Vomica, Silica

Bruised, battered, sore – Arnica, Coffea, Nux Vomica, Rhus Tox

Excruciating, violent – Belladonna, Silica

Throbbing, beating, hammering, pulsating – Aconite, Argentum Nitricum, Belladonna, Nux Vomica, Pulsatilla, Silica

Eyes

- Discharges – Calc Carb, Nat Mur, Nux Vomica, Pulsatilla
- Inflamed – Aconite, Apis, Arnica, Calc Carb, Pulsatilla, Sepia, Silica, Sulphur
- Itching – Calc Carb, Pulsatilla, Rhus Tox, Sulphur

Ears

- Earache – Belladonna, Chamomilla, Phosphorus, Pulsatilla, Sulphur

Nose

- Nosebleed – Aconite, Phosphorus, Sulphur
- Runny – Belladonna, Nat Mur, Phosphorus
- Blocked – Arsenicum, Calc Carb, Nux Vomica

Mouth

- Toothache – Aconite, Chamomilla, Coffea, Sepia

Throat

- Sore throat
  Burning – Aconite, Nat Mur
  On swallowing – Arsenicum, Belladonna, Coffea

Chest

- Asthma (mild) – Aconite, Ipecacuana, Pulsatilla, Silica, Spongia

Back

- Backache – Belladonna, Calc Carb, Graphites, Nat Mur, Nux Vomica, Rhus Tox, Phosphorus

Tummy/Stomach

- Indigestion – Calc Carb, Nux Vomica, Sulphur
  After starchy food – Nat Mur
  After coffee – Nux Vomica
  After grief – Ignatia
  After vexation (being annoyed, frustrated or worried) – Chamomilla

Bladder

- Cystitis
  After sexual intercourse – Staphisagria
  Frequent, burning urination – Apis
  Painful, violent burning – Cantharis
- Incontinence in bed – Arnica, Belladonna, Nat Mur

Rectum

- Constipation – Apis, Calc Carb, Coffea, Nat Mur, Nux Vomica
  Ineffectual urging and straining – Aconite, Calc Carb, Pulsatilla
  Alternating with diarrhoea – Nux Vomica
  Painful – Nat Mur

- Diarrhoea – Aconite, Arsenicum, Phosphorus, Sulphur
  After alcoholic drinks – Nux Vomica
  After beer – Sulphur
  After coffee – Ignatia
  In children – Chamomilla

Male

- Sexual passion
  Diminished – Aconite, Silica
  Increased – Nux Vomica, Phosphorus

Female

- Menses, suppressed – Belladonna, Lachesis, Pulsatilla, Silica
  From emotion – Cimicifuga
  From grief – Ignatia
- Menopause – Lachesis, Sepia
- Period pains – Belladonna, Chamomilla, Nux Vomica, Pulsatilla

Extremities

- Hands
  Arthritic – Calc Carb
- Legs
  Leg cramps in bed – Nux Vomica
- Feet
  Profuse, sweaty feet – Silica
  In-growing toenails – Silica

Skin

Keep in mind when using Homeopathy for a skin condition you will have a much better, long-lasting result, if you treat the condition constitutionally by seeing a Homeopath in person.

- Acne – Belladonna, Sulphur
- Allergic rashes – Apis, Urtica, Rhus Tox, Pulsatilla, Sulphur
- Boils – Arnica, Belladonna, Sulphur

The next section is for general complaints.

Bruises – Arnica
Colds – Aconite to start, then use Nat Mur if nose gets really runny
Fatigue – Phosphorus
Fever – Belladonna
Grazes – Calendula
Hangover – Nux Vomica
Hay fever – Pulsatilla
Indigestion – Nux Vomica

Eczema

I have included this small section on eczema as I have treated so many cases/clients and also have suffered from it myself.

According to Black's Medical Dictionary, eczema is the lay term for dermatitis. Symptoms typically include itching, dryness or cracking and, occasionally, soreness of the skin.

Atopic dermatitis characteristically occurs from ages 3 months to 16 years old, in those with a personal or family history of hay fever, allergic rhinitis or asthma.

Contact allergic dermatitis results from direct contact with a toxic irritant such as bleach, detergents, solvents or lanolin and in extreme cases perfume, nickel jewellery and/or other allergens.

Hahnemann was very averse to treating itchy skin conditions with topical applications or creams. He said that these skin conditions should be treated 'by a thorough internal cure of the whole of this disease' and not by

> violent internal and external remedies, with sharp purgatives...with the Jasser ointment...with solutions of acetate of Lead, with the sublimate of Mercury or sulphate of Zinc, but especially with anointment prepared of fat with Flowers of Sulphur or with the preparation of Mercury; with which they likely and carelessly destroy the eruption...[1]

Jasser ointment was made of sulphate of zinc, now called zinc sulphate, and is used as a herbicide/pesticide to control moss. The side-effects are numerous: nausea, metallic taste, stomach ache, vomiting, and bloody diarrhoea. Breathing in zinc sulphate can irritate the respiratory tract, cause nausea, vomiting, stomach ache, dizziness, depression, metallic taste in the mouth, and death. Exposure by skin contact can damage the skin, leading to ulcers, blisters and scarring. Zinc sulphate can cause severe eye irritation, resulting in redness and pain.

Mercury can still, to this day, be used as a 'treatment' for skin conditions. Topical mercury preparations are still listed in several pharmacopoeias, including those of the USA, UK and several other European countries. It is a severely poisonous substance and can cause nephrotic syndrome, kidney failure, peripheral neuropathy, severe skin irritation, and worse. There has been an alert to remove it from retail sale or prescribed by doctors but it's still available online. Beware! It is very dangerous stuff!

What Hahnemann observed was, even though the skin eruption might have been removed, the patient developed worse symptoms, chronic diseases, and generally reduced their health and well-being. That's if they didn't actually die from some of the treatments used.

My advice would be the same as Samuel's. Don't suppress a skin complaint. Deal with the internal causes, which could be emotional or mental or even spiritual.

I've treated far too many cases of 'eczema' that presented with itchy skin, when really the client was suffering from eating-the-wrong-foods, stressing-about-work/relationship/children or drinking-too-much alcohol or coffee.

Avoiding the stresses and treating the eczema as an 'internal' complaint, not an 'external', brings much longer-lasting and holistic results.

Chapter Ten

Emotional Disturbances
with Suggested Remedies

I wish I'd known about Homeopathy when I was a teen. I might have had a much less stressful time. Homeopathy could have helped my emotional state, as for most of the time from about my late teens to my late twenties I was what could only be described as emotionally 'All Over the Place'.

Now, if I feel an emotional burden I can't shake off, I'll either self-prescribe or visit my Homeopath.

Super!

If you're male, I don't want you to skip this chapter and think that emotions are only something females 'suffer' from. That's just not true! Men have feelings too and, just like women, they need to feel safe, secure and loved.

Here's what one young man in his thirties told me in his first consultation. Gareth works as a supervisor for a building company. He's married and his wife was pregnant with their first child.

I always ask clients what they'd like help with the most, and this is how he replied: 'I'm suffering from stress, anxiety, depression, headaches, frustrated about sex, feelings of guilt, letting people down, dwelling on past mistakes and past regrets.'

He had a complex family with two half-sisters and a half-brother by his mother (as his mother remarried) and an older brother and stepbrother by his father (who also remarried). His father had an affair and left the matrimonial home and disappeared when he was 7. His mother found another partner and he was 'over the moon' that he had a 'new dad'.

But things soured as his new stepdad and his mum worked long hours running their own cleaning business and he had to manage alone, look after his younger siblings, keep house *and* do his school work.

He managed to bury all of his feelings and get married, but when his wife became pregnant with their first child all the anxiety he had suffered as a child resurfaced, hence his appointment with me.

Worry and stress can cause all sorts of feelings to rise and Homeopathy is brilliant at stopping some awful feelings in their tracks.

Emotional Symptoms

Emotional symptoms are feeling angry, sad, weepy, moody, gloomy, over-excited, or sentimental.

You might need emotional help when all you can do is cry, or you well up when someone asks you how you are. Emotional problems include feeling tearful, feeling angry, sighing a lot, not wanting to be on your own, needing company, *not* wanting company and wanting to be on your own, needing hugs and other tactile contact, or randomly sleeping with anyone and everyone you meet.

Keeping a journal and recording your feelings assists greatly when you are in a totally wobbly place. Writing every morning about the things that are upsetting you will allow you to get those feelings 'off your chest'. Being able to talk to someone who has no personal relationship to you will also allow you to untangle these feelings, so book in a counselling session.

Cut Out Coffee

One thing I'd definitely recommend to people that are overly emotional is to cut out coffee completely. Free yourself from the eternal ups and downs that coffee can bring. Start by drinking decaf for 2 weeks, then on the third week have no coffee at all.

You will find by now, amazingly, your emotional ups and downs will have completely reduced.

However, you might find that this seems boring and nothing is going on. Ignore that type of thinking, as it will only send you back to drinking coffee again and being up and down again.

Fine Line

There are degrees of acceptable emotional feelings before they slip into mental health issues. Crying for longer than a few minutes at a time means you are suffering from something psychological. And if you were to cry each and every day for hours and hours, that would be pathological.

However, feeling weepy when you watch a sad film isn't pathological.

I suppose most emotional issues exist because of relationship problems, but you could get equally emotional about a pet or a situation at work. It can be quite tricky untangling where an emotion is coming from as sometimes issues can have been going on for so long you become overwhelmed.

Dr Edward Bach, who developed the Bach Flower Remedies, was a firm believer that 'the Herbs heal our fears, our anxieties, our worries, our faults and our failings, it is these we must seek, and then the disease, no matter what it is, will leave us.'[1]

I completely agree with these sentiments. If we can remove the worries and upsetments that a person feels, then it might just ping them into a much better frame of mind and a better state of health. I'd much rather be happy and 'suffering' from some medical condition than unhappy and physically 'fit'.

Emotional Stability

Getting into a place of emotional stability is an absolute must if we want to feel content and happy with life. Unfortunately, there are plenty of things that can cause us tons of worry, send our blood pressure sky high, cause us anger, fear and grief, and make our lives miserable. Choosing a good remedy early enough will help prevent a downward spiral of ill health and unhappiness.

Homeopaths have been aware of this for centuries. In 1842 Samuel wrote that mental and emotional diseases could be caused by 'faulty upbringing, bad habits, perverted morality, neglect of the spirit, superstitions or ignorance.'[2] In these cases they could be relieved by 'understanding, well-intentioned exhortations, consolation, or with earnest and rational expostulations.'[2]

However, if the emotional upsetment is 'based on a somatic (of the body, not of the mind) disease', then it will just get worse with such treatment and the 'melancholic patient will become still more downcast, plaintive, disconsolate and withdrawn.'[2]

Dr Margery G Blackie, a wonderfully dedicated Homeopath who was appointed physician to the Queen in 1969, wrote in her *The Patient, Not the Cure* in 1976 about a weepy 10-year-old patient of hers:

> There was the case of a little girl of ten who was doing very badly at school and was altogether rather miserable. She had a teacher who was always telling her she could do better, or that she did not try hard enough, and she would often arrive home in tears. She was a great worrier; she fretted over her work, about anyone who was ill in the street where she lived, or some injustice that she had seen. Weeping she would tell her family about it and probably repeat it several times. Her elder sister refused to sleep in the same room because she talked to herself about all her troubles and some nights awoke screaming from nightmares, and then would describe these to anyone who would listen...She was given *Calcarea carbonica* 10m, and did not need to return to the doctor for a year. By then she had skipped a form and was second in her school examinations. She is now grown up and has done well in her work and life.[3]

Now compare this case to Gareth's and you'll understand how treating early, and being aware of and helping someone's emotions, while they're happening, can prevent years of emotional trauma.

Homeopathy can even help extreme emotional trauma. I have treated clients who have been sexually abused in childhood. A good Homeopathic prescription makes all the difference and allows clients to come to a place of peace about their trauma. It doesn't take the memory away but allows 'Life to Go On', and for the person to pick themselves up and carry on. I'm not suggesting you treat something extreme at home. Be sensible; seek help if circumstances are violent or abusive.

If your emotional state doesn't get better from having a good cry or a short walk, eating sensible food, being with your friends or family or having a hug, then think about using the following remedies to help yourself or your loved one:

Calc Carb – Apprehensive, worse towards evening, fears loss of reason, misfortune, contagious diseases. Forgetful, confused, low-spirited. Averse to work or exertion.

Ignatia – Changeable moods, introspective, silently brooding. Melancholic, sad, tearful. Not communicative. Sighing and sobbing. After shocks, grief, disappointment.

Lycopodium – Melancholy, afraid to be alone. Little things annoy. Extremely sensitive. Averse to undertaking new things. Loss of self-confidence. Constant fear of breaking down under stress. Weak memory, confused thoughts. Sadness in morning on waking.

Nat Mur – Diseases caused by thinking too much, ill effects of grief, fright, anger etc. Depressed, particularly in chronic diseases. Consolation aggravates. Wants to be alone to cry. Tears with laughter. Irritable, gets into a passion about trifles.

Pulsatilla – Weeps easily. Timid, irresolute. Fears in evening to be alone. Fears the dark and ghosts. Likes sympathy. Children like fuss and caresses. Easily discouraged. Morbid dread of the opposite sex. Religious melancholy. Given to extremes of pleasure and pain. Highly emotional. Mentally an April day.

Sepia – Indifferent to those loved best. Averse to occupation, to family. Irritable, easily offended. Dreads to be alone. Very sad. Weeps when telling symptoms. Anxious towards evening, indolent.

Chapter Eleven

Mental Problems with Suggested Remedies

I thought long and hard before I included this chapter as there is an idea that 'only' psychiatrists can treat mental conditions. While it is true that mental health professionals see and treat a wide range of mental conditions, they almost certainly can only treat the person when some long-sounding name or label has been given to them.

Yes, there certainly are conditions such as bipolar and schizophrenia, but you won't find a psychiatrist diagnosing: 'been abandoned by mother syndrome' or 'bullied at school by older girls disease' or 'financially struggling while bringing up three children ailment' or 'working long relentless hours for never satisfied boss disorder'.

As I mentioned earlier, Homeopaths treat people, not diseases, so their treatment is more likely to 'fit' the patient, rather than trying to squash the patient's diagnosis onto their psyche. I also think it's important to always hear the person's 'story' as it will give me an idea of if they're likely to recover, or if, in their story-telling, they might be telling themselves that they're incurable. I must also point out that serious mental health issues will not respond to one dose of a remedy. A severe case of mental health unwellness will need a team of people not only treating the mental state but also supporting the person in other ways such as with housing or job hunting. Unlike having a physical complaint, mental problems are not visible and most people are fearful of not only other people having mental health issues, but also treating them, supporting them and helping them.

Support groups are good when a person has reached a little further down the line of recovery.

My thoughts are we need to change the way people with

mental illness are helped, as the drugs don't always work.

As a Homeopath I have experience of dealing with mental illness not only in my private practice but also in a drugs detox centre where I worked with another Homeopath for 8 years. We met and helped numbers of seriously unwell people. We should be empowering the mentally ill, not disempowering them with cocktails of chemicals.

If you break your leg, no-one gives you something that changes the way you think for the worse. Tranquillisers and antidepressants alter people's perceptions, alter their sleeping and alter their appetite. The list goes on.

The focus would be better spent on helping people with mental illness eat sensibly, have exercise every day, spend less time on computers (biggest cause of mental upsetment: too much screen time). Help them learn how to relax, learn how to breathe, do yoga. The alternatives are there...

It would be far more helpful if mental illness was prevented by keeping an eye on these important factors:

- Diet
- Exercise
- Stress

Someone who spends weeks at a time under stressful conditions is going to 'live' more in their heads than their body, which results in unhealthy thinking, which causes unhealthy lifestyle choices, which can then cause mental breakdowns.

The key things to look out for are:

- Lack of sleep: not enough sleep, late nights, persistent insomnia can all contribute to mental breakdown.
- Bad eating: too much caffeine, too much sugar, irregular meals or lack of food. Homelessness and starvation can seriously alter the way you think.

- Lack of fresh air: too much time spent indoors or using computers or electrical equipment.
- Isolation: no friends or family.
- Too much brain work: university students are at special risk of spending too much time studying, drinking alcohol, living irregular hours, lacking in sleep and frequently suffer mental problems. This includes people studying for exams, or tests, or people that do repetitive task jobs in confined places with no access to fresh air, like factory work, data entry or call-centre work.
- Unemployment can also lead to mental health problems, as being indoors all day with no access to fresh air and sunlight can make people moody and morose.

Liberation from Thought

Without thought we are liberated.

I will give you an example.

Imagine that you go for a short walk, down a country lane through a few trees. As you're walking you could very easily spend your whole journey thinking about who said what, what you'd like to say, what you didn't say, what went wrong...the lists can be endless.

What if you tackled it another way?

What if you had this short walk down a country lane and through a few trees and instead you *fully experienced everything* as it happens.

Do you hear the rustle of the trees' leaves?

Do you feel the hard-baked earth underneath your shoes?

Do you see the different-coloured flowers growing by the side of the path?

You could also experience the breeze that might be blowing through your hair.

Just spending 10 minutes, in any given day, experiencing everything around you *as it happens* can liberate you from anxious or troubling thoughts.

An even easier version of this is to concentrate on your breathing.

Breath Counting

If you get stuck into a completely negative frame of mind, breathe in and out and, as you breathe, count from 1 to 10.

Breathe in – 1
Breathe out – 2
Breathe in – 3
Breathe out – 4

And so on until you reach 10. Then when you get to 10 go back to 1 again and breathe in on the count of 1.

Mental Help

When your mental symptoms include irrational thoughts, having extreme highs and lows, feeling out of control, sleeplessness, great fear and anxiety and a disregard of your physical circumstances, you are in need of help.

You might be homeless, threatened with homelessness, out of work, or in a bad relationship. Don't wait until you completely lose the plot, because someone is likely to alert the authorities and, worst-case scenario, you are sectioned and admitted to a mental health treatment centre.

Before you seek help, make a note of what is worrying you the most and on a piece of paper write what you'd like to have happen, not your fears.

You might write something like 'I would like my obsessive compulsive disorder to be less of a worry.'

Or you might write: 'I would like to stop thinking about scary things like dying.'

Most people when they have a problem are likely to ask their friends or family for advice, but this is the one time when, unless they work in psychiatric care, they are unlikely to be able to help you.

The reason is they have no experience of mental problems and while their help might be well intentioned, they've never been with someone mentally unstable or seen how things can progress or equally how things *can* improve with the right help.

You wouldn't expect your friends to understand bungee jumping if they'd never done it before, so don't expect them to understand mental health problems.

The sort of help you need is from someone experienced in mental health issues.

If you are already on a treatment programme and are not happy with your care, get in touch with the organisations listed below and see if you can get a second opinion.

In my opinion some drugs are worse than the problems they are supposed to solve. If the side-effects of drugs that you are already on are affecting your day-to-day existence, this is the time to have a review.

In the UK the help offered to people with mental health issues is extremely mixed, complex and founded on issues of control and authority. These obviously are not helpful foundations to assist a mental health recovery.

You are better off seeking help from a self-help group and there are a number run by Mind.

UK:

- http://www.mind.org.uk/help/mind_in_your_area
- http://www.sane.org.uk/

USA:

- http://www.mentalhealthamerica.net/go/find_support_group

Online self-help groups can be counter-intuitive and might drag you further into the mental problems you have already. So be careful about the online self-help groups you join. Try not to spend too much time using your computer. A short, brisk walk in the fresh air will benefit you far more than 2 hours 'discussing' your fears with someone you'll never meet.

Chemical Poisoning

You might find that your whole life needs a total review. You might need to reduce or cut out stimulants, coffee, alcohol, cigarettes or other forms of chemical poisoning.

The way of life advocated by Rudolf Steiner is the way to go. He founded a form of healthy lifestyle that supports the person, and the planet, called Anthroposophy.

- UK http://www.anthroposophy.org.uk/
- USA http://www.anthroposophy.org/

These groups have doctors trained in Homeopathy and gentle forms of treatment and if you can find yourself an Anthroposophic doctor you're less likely to be prescribed drugs.

- UK http://www.ahasc.org.uk/health/anthroposophic-health care/doctors.aspx
- USA http://www.paam.net/home.html

I'm not suggesting that you become a total hippie and live in a yurt, but spending more time in the quiet, or in beautiful solitary places, will give your thoughts a chance to calm down.

If you would like NHS Homeopathic treatment, and you live in the UK, you can get an appointment by asking your GP for a referral to one of the Homeopathic hospitals which are based in London, Bristol, Liverpool and Glasgow:

http://www.britishhomeopathic.org/getting_treatment/homeo

pathy_in_the_nhs/

In the UK Homeopathy is divided into private treatments by practitioners trained in Homeopathy (like me) or doctors who are trained in medicine, then train postgrad in Homeopathy, and then practise in the NHS.

UK practitioners can register with various organisations; there is no one place for all of them but this site lists some helpful info: http://www.findahomeopath.org.uk/

Or you could search for one with the Federation of Holistic Therapists. I'm a member of this organisation and you can search on their website here: http://findatherapist.fht.org.uk/

This UK charity also has useful information: http://www. homeopathyactiontrust.org/

- Worldwide info: http://nationalcenterforhomeopathy.org/
- Europe: http://www.homeopathy-ecch.org/
- Switzerland: http://liga.iwmh.net/

Homeopathy is Brilliant for Mental Health Issues
Why?

Because over the years Homeopaths have built up an enormous body of knowledge on the way people think, because it's our thinking that gets us into trouble.

Thinking that people are out to get you, or that neighbours are planning your destruction, or thinking that your boss hates you or your boyfriend doesn't like you...all these thoughts will easily push a person into a state of mental unwellness.

In the Homeopathic provings, plenty of weird and wonderful mental symptoms have been uncovered and if you can think of a really weird thought, there will be someone somewhere who has also thought the same.

Homeopaths don't really talk about this much. It's sort of accepted that the most important part of 'taking someone's case' is getting an understanding of their mental processes.

Random Driver

I treated a lady a few years ago who randomly drove her car around and ended up at someone's house and walked into the house and waited for her family to join her (which they didn't as they didn't know she was there, but she thought in her confused state that they did).

I analysed her case using the rubrics from the Repertory:

Travel, desire to
Home, desires to go
Homesickness

In the Materia Medica the remedy I gave her is listed as: 'Always wants to go somewhere, when away from home, wants to go there and when there, wants to go somewhere else'.

She was stuck between wanting to go out, but when she was out wanting to get back home. Her husband was very worried about her, and went to fetch her, and when she came to see me her rational self was a little wobbly. After a long amount of listening to her case, I discovered the reason for her strange behaviour, which was to do with an enormous fear from sexual abuse in her childhood.

Now, that's not to say that all fears from childhood will make someone want to go out, then want to come home again. Similar circumstances don't produce the same symptoms in people. That's an important consideration in Homeopathy.

All we need to know is how the person is feeling now, and how their Vital Force is expressing it.

Are they shuffling around the house or moving in their chair, are they muttering to themselves or flicking imaginary fluff off their clothes?

These are all small things we might not notice if we're too busy giving someone a 'diagnosis'.

Homeopathy doesn't need a diagnosis; it cares about the

person's *expression* of their inner state.

Sleep

There is one thing that's critical to good mental health, and that's sleep. Not enough of us have it or experience it and, like a fleeting day of good weather, as soon as it appears, it can go away again. Good sleep is so important to your mental health, never mind your physical health, so do make sure you do all you can to make it better.

Here are some responses to the question 'How is your sleep?' in a BBC survey:[1]

Janice

My sleep patterns were disrupted because of the night shifts I worked as a nurse some 30 odd years ago. I worked then and now (not as a nurse) I might add, on max 4 hours sleep. If my sleep is disturbed that is it. Used to stress me out. I was on prescribed drugs for sleep for some time and when my GP wanted me to cut down on it, I gave it up and nowadays I just try to relax instead of stressing.

Gregor

I've had disturbed sleep for about 6 months. Every night I drop off easily, then wake up every 1–2 hours. Tried all advice, short of benzodiazepines, to no avail.

Christina

I developed auto-immune diseases as a direct result of sleep deprivation. I will always have these and they will not go away. I was fit and healthy before suffering the sleep loss, so I know first-hand what this can do to a person's body. Some nights I only got 4 hours' sleep due to banging and stamping and shouting from the flat above. Sustained over time this does real damage.

You will be pleased to know Homeopaths have been recording people's sleep for hundreds of years and analysing data from provers and have built up a massive directory of sleeping issues. From A to Z there are symptoms, from people being anxious *about* sleep to yawning *from* lack of sleep and due to dreams, being disturbed *by* hunger, menses and even visions.

I don't have room here to list all the different possibilities and types of sleep deprivation, but do keep in mind that sleep is very important to your mental health.

Sleep Journal

First thing you need to decide, if you're going to help yourself, is what is causing your sleeplessness?

Are you sleepless or just lacking in good sleep?

Keep a dream and sleep journal for at least a week. It's no good saying you've got a sleep problem if you can't describe it in any way or you're not too sure exactly what the problem is. With good Homeopathic treatment the more specific you can be, the better your treatment can be tailored to your individual problem.

You will need to record, daily, what time you went to bed, what you did before you went to bed, who you sleep with (if at all) and how they might have affected your sleep, and how you are feeling or felt during the day.

Rate yourself on a scale of 1 to 10; 10 being really good and 1 being bad.

So, if you had an overall bad day because your boss shouted at you, you missed your train, your partner/friend didn't reply to your texts, and you felt depressed by the time you went to bed, then rate yourself 2/10.

Give each day a rating. Then you can see if your sleep fluctuates according to how your day is rated.

Record also what time you woke and briefly how you felt when you woke and, most importantly, any dreams you may have had.

People that have never kept a sleep journal will find the whole process rather intimidating to start with. Don't let that put you off; one week in your life is a small amount of time to spend on helping you get good sleep and improve your mental state of mind.

Use a journal you like, use a pen that writes easily, and keep your journal BY THE BED.

Now, let's divide your symptoms into the following:

Find out if any foods have caused your lack of sleep. Too much coffee or tea? Eating too late? Eating heavy food for dinner?

If any outside circumstances, such as noise outside your bedroom, have affected you.

If any personal stresses are causing it, such as a relationship break-up, family loss, house move, job change, birth or death of someone.

Is it caused by or affected by your work?

Maybe the temperature or the weather is affecting your sleep. Are you cold? Or hot? Or is your room damp or cold? Is your duvet the wrong tog? The bed too soft or hard? Is your pillow comfortable? All of these will affect your sleep.

Or is it nothing you can place?

Change the Things You Can Change

Now that you've kept your journal for one week, change the things you can change:

- Get a new duvet, or pillow.
- Eat or drink less of the foods that are causing the problem.
- TIDY YOUR BEDROOM!

When I ask people to describe their bedroom, what's in it and the state of their sleeping area, I find a lot of the time the bedroom is cluttered with sleep-preventing equipment such as TVs, DVDs, computers, iPods, iPhones, iPads and various other electrical equipment!

You do NOT need your mobile phone in your bedroom or anywhere near you while you sleep, unless you're camping.

Since your body not only runs on your breath and your heart circulation, it also uses teeny electrical pulses to move bits here and there. Your nervous system sends messages from your brain to your foot to move it, or your hand to pick something up. Having a bedroom with too much electrical equipment can and might very possibly interfere with your own electrical system. The only pieces of electrical equipment that should be in your bedroom on a permanent basis are lights, heating and, if you're very sensitive to pollution, an ioniser.

Also, if you have 'things' under the bed, move them to another room.

If your bedroom is full of furniture, ask yourself, do you really need ALL of it? Do you need boxes of 'stuff' or lots of other bits and bobs? Having a really good clear-out, just in itself, will improve your sleep 100%.

Is your bedroom tidy? And funnily enough, is your living room tidy? I can't tell you the amount of times my family's sleep has been deprived because the living room was left in a mess.

Tidy up as much as you can before you go to sleep and if you find you've got too many 'things' to tidy up, take them to the charity shop or throw them away.

Bed Room

Your bedroom should contain:

A bed…

And lots of…

Room.

Having space in your bedroom will bring space into your mind, especially if it's cluttered with worry and anxiety.

If you are truly finding it hard to throw things away or tidy up, then I would recommend you have one dose of Sulphur 30c before you start.

Other Things You Can Change

Other things you can change are your eating habits and your caffeine intake. Stress causes people to either eat loads or stop eating altogether. Make an attempt to alter these.

You can also change the way you feel about things by writing the situation or the person a letter and burning the letter.

Obviously you can't change your work hours too easily, but if your job is causing you too much stress then it would only be sensible to start looking for another job.

If you've just broken up with someone, you can't change that, but you can change how you deal with it. In addition to taking a relevant remedy, you could again write the person a letter, this time putting all your feelings into the letter and ending it with the things that upset you the most, and what you would have liked to have done differently. Burn the letter safely over the sink or in a metal tray and either put the ashes into the bin or, if you're more romantic, let them loose in some wind, or bury them in a pretty or remote location, or add some pieces to running water such as a stream or river. Be careful not to cause damage to the elements, by using a small amount only. Put the remainder in the bin.

Here are some remedy classifications. If you'd like to see these listings in more detail, they are in Kent's Repertory.[2]

Sleep

- Disturbed – Aconite, Graphites, Sulphur
  By dreams – Aconite, Ignatia, Nat Mur, Nux Vomica
  By hunger – Ignatia
- Interrupted
  By thirst – Nat Mur

- Restless – Aconite, Belladonna, Pulsatilla, Rhus Tox, Sulphur
- Sleeplessness – Arsenicum, Chamomilla, Coffea, Lachesis, Nux Vomica, Phosphorus, Rhus Tox, Sepia, Silicea, Sulphur
  From anxiety – Arnica, Arsenicum, Belladonna, Nat Mur, Nux Vomica
  From coldness – Arsenicum, Calc Carb, Graphites, Nat Mur, Nux Vomica, Phosphorus
  From coldness of feet – Phosphorus
  From excitement – Coffea, Nux Vomica
  From grief – Ignatia, Nat Mur
  From hunger – Ignatia, Phosphorus
  During her period/menstruation – Ignatia, Nat Mur
  After mental strain – Nux Vomica
  From slight noise – Nux Vomica, Phosphorus
  From shocks – Arsenicum, Nat Mur, Phosphorus
  From thoughts/activity of mind – Arsenicum, Calc Carb, Coffea, Nux Vomica, Pulsatilla. Same idea always repeated – Coffea, Graph, Pulsatilla
  After tobacco – Nux Vomica
  From weariness – Arnica
  After wine – Coffea, Nux Vomica

Homeopathic Mental Stress Remedies

The Homeopathic remedies that will help with mental stress are:

Aconite (also called Aconitum Napellus) – For great fear, anxiety and/or physical and mental restlessness, fright. Forebodings and fears. Fears death but believes that he will soon die, predicts the day. Fears the future, a crowd, crossing the street. Restlessness, tossing about. Tendency to start. Imagination acute, clairvoyance. Music is unbearable, makes them sad. Thinks their thoughts come from the stomach – that parts of his body are abnormally thick. Feels as if what had just been done was a dream.

Argentum Nitricum (Nitrate of Silver) – For fear, anxiety and/or apprehension regarding future events. Thinks their understanding will and must fail. Fearful and nervous, impulse to jump out of the window. Faintish and tremulous. Melancholic, apprehension of serious disease. Time passes too slowly. Memory weak. Errors of perception. Impulsive, wants to do things in a hurry. Peculiar mental impulses. Fears and anxieties and hidden irrational motives for actions.

Arsenicum Album – For great anguish and feeling restless. Changes place continually. Fears, of death, of being left alone. Great fear, with cold sweat. Thinks it useless to take medicine. Suicidal. Despair drives them from place to place. Sensitive to disorder and confusion.

Aurum Metallicum (Gold) – For deep gloom and despair and wanting to commit suicide. Feeling of self-condemnation and utter worthlessness. Profound despondency, with thorough disgust of life, and thoughts of suicide. Talks of committing suicide. Great fear of death. Fear of people. Mental derangements. Constant rapid questioning without waiting for reply. Cannot do things fast enough. Oversensitiveness, to noise, excitement, confusion.

Hyoscyamus – Very suspicious. Talkative, obscene, lascivious mania, uncovers body, jealous, foolish. Great hilarity, inclined to laugh at everything. Delirium, with attempt to run away. Low, muttering speech, constant lint picking of bedding and clothes, deep stupor.

Ignatia – For mental stress and strain from shock, bereavement and fright.

Lachesis – Great loquacity (talkativeness). Amative. Sad in the morning, no desire to mix with the world. Restless and uneasy, does not wish to attend to business, wants to be off somewhere all the time. Jealous. Suspicious. Nightly delusion of fire. Religious insanity. Derangement of the time sense.

Nux Vomica – For feeling extremely irritable, fiery temperament and/or impatient. Sensitive to all impressions. Ugly, malicious. Cannot bear noises, odours, light etc. Does not want to be touched. Time passes too slowly. Disposed to reproach others. Sullen, fault-finding.

Phosphorus – For feeling extremely sensitive, fearing being alone, of thunderstorms, fear of the dark, disease and death. Great lowness of spirits. Easily vexed. Fearfulness, as if something were creeping out of every corner. Clairvoyant state. Great tendency to start. Loss of memory. Paralysis of the insane. Dread of death when alone. Brain feels tired. Insanity, with an exaggerated idea of one's own importance. Excitable. Restless. Fidgety. Hypo-sensitive, indifferent.

Sulphur – Very forgetful. Difficult thinking. Delusions, thinks rags are beautiful, thinks that he is immensely wealthy. Busy all the time. Irritable. Affections spoiled, destroyed. Very selfish, no regard for others. Religious melancholy. Averse to business, loafs about. Too lazy to rouse himself. Imagining giving wrong thing to people, causing their death. Irritable, depressed, thin and weak, even with a good appetite.

Potency

Severe or worrying mental conditions respond best to high potencies. Start with a 30c. Repeat every hour while in acute state. Don't go on longer than a week without asking for further help. You might need to get to 200c or higher to feel any benefit, but if you have to go higher it's best to consult a professional Homeopath.

Chapter Twelve

Spiritual Difficulties
with Suggested Remedies

Due to the nature of my work, I do see numbers of people that have reached a spiritual crisis. It's the sort of thing I am happy to discuss with them. Were you to go to your doctor and tell him you've reached a crisis in your spirituality, you're likely to get a referral to a psychiatrist. Even fewer people discuss life's bigger questions with priests, simply because the levels of dogma are so high and the entry fee so expensive. Weekly attendance at mass or church isn't appealing to everyone.

In a fast world, who has time to think about their reason for living?

How many people worry about their soul while they're running for a bus or having a pint in the pub? When you're busy, existential questions get put on the back burner. But when someone you know dies, it can make you question lots of things.

Generally it's the death of someone you know that makes you question your own existence.

The questions I get asked a lot are:

- Why am I here?
- What is my Life Purpose?
- Why did I get ill?

Sometimes people are just beginning their journey into spirituality; sometimes they've been hard at work for a number of years and have reached a plateau, or worse, have ground to a halt.

So what is spirituality?

The dictionary definition is: 'of or concerned with the spirit'.

And what is the spirit?

'Person's animating principle or intelligence, person's soul, disembodied person or incorporeal being...' Incorporeal: 'without substance or material existence'.

So we're not talking about something that we can actually feel or experience in the same way as drinking a glass of water.

Since so few people even admit to following a religion and prefer to classify themselves as 'spiritual', when they hit a crisis there is less ability to find help.

Ah...but Homeopathy has already covered this. Questions like 'Why am I here?' and other philosophical questions have been asked by numerous provers and Homeopaths for hundreds of years, so we can more easily help those clients.

Hahnemann not only was a pragmatist, practically sorting out his patients' conditions; he also had what we would now call a 'spiritual side' and was at great pains to talk about it in his *Organon of the Medical Art*:

> The Life Force in Health and Disease
> #9 In the healthy human state, the spirit-like life force that enlivens the material organism as dynamis, governs without restriction and keeps all parts of the organism in admirable, harmonious, vital operation, as regards both feelings and functions, so that our indwelling, rational spirit can freely avail itself of this living, healthy instrument for the higher purposes of our existence.[1]

The modern translation of this reads:

> In health, the life force keeps all parts of the organism in harmony.

Life Force

In Homeopathic colleges we learn about a thing called the Vital Force. That part of us that keeps us connected to something eternal. The Chinese call it *Chi* or *Qi*; other cultures call it *Prana,* *Cit, Mana* or *Ruah.* It's not something you can touch or see. You can't find it by dissecting a rat. You won't find it in a test tube or in a Petri dish. All living things possess it. It's not measurable. You can't have more or less of it; it just 'is'.

I don't actually think we can gain more of it by praying or going to church. It's with us during our lives and until our death. It exists inside and without us.

Permanently.

The English language is so lacking in allowing us to even write about it and we have to resort to words like Soul or Spirit or Essence. You either know what it is, or you don't, and I won't try and describe it any further. I'm sure there are plenty of writers who have. I'm not one of them.

In Wenda Brewster O'Reilly's wonderful translation of *The Organon* she explains Hahnemann's use of the word soul:

Intermediary between the spirit and the emotional mind...Hahnemann indicates that the soul has feelings and volition. He states, 'It appears as if the soul of the patient feels, with exasperation and sadness, the truth of these rational expostulations and acts directly upon the body as if it wanted to restore the harmony that has been lost...'

In #229 he refers to the 'indignant soul languishing in the fetters of a sick body.'

In #225–227 Hahnemann discusses diseases which are spun and maintained by the soul.

In #228 he discusses the diet of the soul, involving the psychologically fitting approach to be taken towards a patient with a mental or emotional disease.[2]

So Hahnemann was in recognition of the fact that human beings have a soul, as well as a mind and a body. Thank goodness for that! We're not just a collection of cells!

In the Repertory we have rubrics such as under

Mind,
Delusions:
– Separated body:
Mind are separate; body and

Soul
Body was too small for the soul, or separated from the soul

Delusions:
– God
He is in communication with God
He is God, then he is the devil
He is in the presence of God
Sees God
He is the object of God's vengeance.[4]

These are really important considerations to help someone who's in a dreadful conflict about their 'soul's welfare'. Obviously we don't expect the answers to these sorts of questions every day of the week, but when a close relative has died, or you've lost a baby or you are suffering from a life-limiting illness, you might question 'why' you're here.

In one of the provings I conducted in 2009 using sand from the Karnak Temple in Egypt, some of the provers had quite enlightening experiences and higher-self connections.

Day 3
Prover 15
6.30pm Talked with supervisor. Made me realise I have done a lot of spiritual work recently – since Saturday in fact.

• Reiki Share, Saturday

- Reiki Share one to one, Monday
- Spiritual book group, Monday
- Wrote piece about connecting to each other in spiritual way for UK Reiki Federation Magazine

Day 15

Prover 5

2pm The remedy seems to make me think that the proving has a spiritual dimension to it – an Eastern approach to life. The idea of acceptance and letting go of the things we can't control, the idea of living in the present – not worrying about the past or the future. Today I have a serendipity I didn't have last week. It's as if all that angry angst I was feeling had chilled out into a more positive way of feeling detached, rather than a selfish way.

One prover struggled with their spirituality and started praying.

Day 13

Prover 9

Lack of sleep and intense pressure I'm under. Don't want to see or talk to anyone, even close family. Daughter worried about me. Told (supervisor) I feel shaky, have palpitations, tightness in chest when talking to the mental health people, have even 'resorted' to praying (which I haven't done for many years) as so desperate about C's lack of care.

Day 22

Have been praying for the first time in many years. Just come to end of 9-day traditional prayer cycle used in Catholic Church to Virgin Mary – have not practised religion for about 40 years.

Some remedies are more in tune with spiritual questions than others. Even in the proving of Arnica, not something you would think of in a spiritual crisis, one of the provers 'prays quietly for (her) soul'.

The remedies I would recommend for questions about Life, The Universe and Everything are Anacardium, Aurum, Calc Carb, Cannabis Indica, Hyoscyamus, Lachesis, Stramonium, Thuja and Veratrum Album:

Anacardium – Thinks he is possessed of two persons or wills. Fixed ideas; that mind and body are separated. Religious mania. Indifference to his religion. Feels as if he has two wills, one commanding him to do what the other forbids.

Aurum – Weeping, praying and self-reproach from heart disease. Weeping, because he imagines he has lost the affection of his friends. Religious mania, imagines herself irretrievably lost.

Calc Carb – Bright little girls 8 or 9 years old who become sad and melancholic and begin to talk about future world and Angels, want to die and go there and want to read the Bible all day.

Cannabis Indica – Lost in delicious thoughts. Can't realise her identity, and chronic vertigo as if floating off. Ecstatic, heavenly.

Hyoscyamus – Talks of imaginary things, but has no wants and makes no complaints. Not a moment quiet, continual calling out that they saw the devil; denies themselves guilty of theft (after being harshly accused of it), or that they have any concern with witches. Constant talking, especially on religious subjects.

Lachesis – Compelling delusions; thinks themselves under superhuman control; thinks they are dead and preparations are being made for their funeral. Ecstasy, and almost prophetic perceptions, all with a vivid imagination. Religious affections; in children. Feels as if they have two wills. Uses exalted language [in a girl, after excessive study].

Stramonium – Devout, earnest, beseeching and ceaseless talking. Loquacious, garrulous, laughing, singing, swearing, praying, rhyming. Sees ghosts, hears voices, talks with spirits. Religious mania. Religious insanity; despair of salvation; inspired talking, singing, pious looks. Young men or women who pray, sing or talk so devoutly or constantly as to excite the sympathy of all in the home. Think they are divine; that they are in communication with God, deliver emphatic sermons, prophecies. Praying at night.

Thuja – Delusion divided into two parts and could not tell which part they had possession on waking. Delusion, fancied body was too small for soul or that it was separated from soul. Anxiety about salvation.

Veratrum Album – Despair about salvation. Imagines the world on fire; prays loudly on knees, believes they are the risen Christ. Delusions; that they are in communication with God; of wealth. Religious affections. Talks much about religious things; prattles about religious subjects and about vows to be performed. Suicidal tendency from religious despair.[2,3]

I'll give you an example of the sort of things that I get asked by email and my remedy recommendation. Maddie is unfortunately talking about how her life will be, *after* she is dead. I take these sorts of hints seriously.

I have always had feelings of clairvoyance, intuitiveness, and a natural knowing of one's future. This issue is I'm a jack-of-all-trades and it's bitter sweet. I am intrigued and successful in a lot of affairs. I now want to be famous for leaving a mark on our Planet before I go. I live by Mother Teresa's: *Spread love everywhere you go. Let no one ever come to you without leaving happier.* I also read people and am usually accurate. I seek out your guidance, thank you :)

Peace and love,

Maddie

She says she is successful but does that sound to you like someone who *feels* successful? Aurum is made from gold. A fitting substance for people wanting to shine. She wants to 'be famous for leaving a mark on our Planet'. This particular remedy is for the person who is: 'duty-bound, workaholic, industrious; always busy and working, never finished'[2] and 'Cheerful while thinking of death'.[3]

She doesn't sound depressed but she's not entirely happy either, otherwise she wouldn't have gone to the trouble to email me. She's concerned about her soul.

This is just a teeny example of how Homeopathy can help in a spiritual crisis and gives you some resources to help yourself or those close to you a little in this area.

Chapter Thirteen

Case Examples

I am going to share with you some cases from my own private practice. These clients or their families have given permission for their cases to be published, which I am extremely thankful for. I am including them, as they are examples of real problems that people come with, that are so different from how conventional medicine views health and disease.

Teen Mental Health

Watching your teen suffer from a mental health issue can be the most excruciating and upsetting experience. Even if you manage to get some professional help within the NHS, you still have to negotiate endless psychiatric visits, probing questions and chemical prescriptions without even dealing with the initial sense of loss of your child's childhood.

Childhood and teen years should be celebrated and can be the most joyous times of life. However, when mental health problems strike, it feels as if your world has fallen apart.

Homeopathy is a form of medical treatment that doesn't interfere with the body's own ability to self-correct. Patients have been suffering from mental health issues since the beginning of time and Homeopaths have a vast array of relevant treatments. They don't produce side-effects or cause mental health issues to worsen.

I have been working in Homeopathic private practice for over 15 years and support my clients during mental-health upsetments.

I use the word 'upsetment' to describe any form of mental imbalance. I do not use words like schizophrenic, bipolar, manic depression or hallucination. All these words form a barrier to true understanding, and relief. In conventional medicine, treatment cannot begin until a diagnosis has been made.

Treatment Starts Right Away

In Homeopathy, treatment can start straight away, as we are interested in symptoms not diagnosis. A diagnosis only helps a practitioner, not the patient. The patient needs treatment, understanding, and space and time to heal.

We negotiate a suitable course of treatment, review it as and when needed, and ensure that the child in question is supported, heard and understood.

Gentle

I have a firm belief that the gentle, non-addictive approach brings speedier and longer-lasting results.

Samuel Hahnemann, the originator of Homeopathy, understood health and illness and was completely at loggerheads with the prevailing peer view that illness is caused by something outside the body. That diseases are caused by a virus, a bacteria, an injury or, as is the classic explanation in mental health, 'a chemical imbalance in the brain'.

If this were truly true, that the brain was chemically imbalanced, then people suffering from mental ill health would be dead.

As Joanna Moncrieff says in her *The Myth of the Chemical Cure: A Critique of Psychiatric Drug Treatment*,[1] professional, commercial and political vested interests have shaped this view. Mental illness has nothing to do with chemicals in the brain but has a lot to do with what preceded the mental upsetment, as Peter Kinderman PhD points out in 'A Psychological Model of Mental Disorder'.[2]

In older children, and those in their teen years, indulging in too many stimulants, alcohol, drugs and cigarettes can cause mental upsetment.

In younger children an erratic lifestyle, grief, loss and uncertainty can also cause mental upsetment.

In my private practice I have seen and treated children with a variety of 'diagnoses'. Everything from ADD, ADHD, bipolar, schizophrenia, anxiety, OCD, personality disorders and depression to eating disorders and various syndromes. I put these diagnoses to one side and ask about the child themselves. In Homoeopathy we want to know all about the person, not the condition, because it is the person that we treat.

Dynamic

Hahnemann said diseases are dynamic, not material.

They come from what we call in Homeopathy an aetiology. This could be a miasm (an inherited susceptibility to something), an emotional experience, or a physical injury that then puts strain on other parts of the body. In Allopathy, or conventional medicine, the emphasis is to identify the cause of the illness, and then remove it. The side-effect of this is to sometimes remove, literally, parts of people's bodies, or to incapacitate various functions of the body.

Let's step back a bit. Health is not just the absence of disease. It is about feeling in the flow, enjoying life, not being held back physically or mentally from achieving goals and desires. Illness isn't something that happens to the body; it is something that the body opens itself to.

You know what it's like, as you've experienced this yourself. A cold is going round at work, and three of your work colleagues out of a total of eight have caught this cold. You, however, are feeling very bright and breezy and are involved in an exciting project. You don't get the cold; in fact you don't get it until you take a long weekend off. If the cold was caused by an outside event, how is it that you didn't catch it when everyone else was succumbing to it? You didn't catch it because your mental health and physical well-being were bigger than the cold itself.

Here are some other examples:

Being Bullied

Your sister, who is three years younger than you, lives in the same house, eats the same food, has the same parents as you, and becomes mentally unwell after a episode of bullying at school. You were bullied at the same age yourself but it never affected your mental health. Why is this? In Homeopathy we call it susceptibility, so when we're treating someone, we're looking at and thinking about their own personal susceptibility.

The Death of His Beloved Pet

Ben came to see me with his mother. He was 16 years old. He had been feeling unwell for 7 months and was anxious, sleepless and lacking in energy. He was also being influenced by different atmospheres and felt ungrounded. His awareness had been heightened and he said he was suffering from 'hyper awareness'. He was also seeing colours around people and when he played the piano different chords were different hues of colours.

He was also over-thinking.

I asked what had happened prior to him feeling unwell, and he told me his dog had died. He had had her for 11 years and they were really close and when Poppy died he felt a part of him had also died. He and Poppy had slept together since he was 6 years old. She used to sleep on the pillow next to him.

As his mother was so worried about Ben's mental health, she had quite rightly taken him to the doctor. However, there are no medical treatments that have been approved for child mental ill-health and he was prescribed a frightening amount of medication that was developed for adults: Prozac, Risperidone, Zopiclone, Valium, Ativan and Amitriptyline.

Needless to say, none of these medications had worked, he had suffered all their side-effects, and was still feeling anxious and sleepless.

I prescribed the Homeopathic remedy Ignatia 30c, one dose before bed for 3 nights, and a new remedy I had proved earlier in the year made from a sample of sand taken from the Karnark Temple in Egypt which helps with loss and bereavement: http://www.maryenglish.com/karnak-temple.html

Six days later his mother phoned me to say that Ben was feeling better. He had had a good cry, mourned the loss of his beloved pet, and had even changed his bedroom around and moved his bed and was now sleeping better.

Seven months of 'conventional' treatment had done nothing to reduce his anxiety.

Six days of Homoeopathic treatment had cured the case...

Ignatia and How to Heal a Broken Heart

Sometimes a complaint is more than meets the eye, and symptoms and general unwellness can date back to a negative occurrence. This is what we call the aetiology of symptoms or more simply 'never-been-well-since'.

The difference between a conventional doctor's treatment for emotional problems, compared to how much Homeopathy can offer, is considerable. Apart from tranquillisers or anti-depressants, conventional medicine is restricted in its ability to help heal the most common emotional complaint for men and women: A Broken Heart.

When a relationship ends, the world seems to end too, but a few doses of this tried and trusted remedy will ensure you're back to your old self and all the anxiety has dissipated. If I had to take one remedy to a desert island, Ignatia would be my unhesitating choice. I have seen more improvements in patients from this one remedy than any other, barring Arnica.

A few years ago I was treating a client who recommended a friend to me. I made a home visit as she was too unwell to leave the house and her energy was seriously down.

Eighteen months previously a relationship had ended. She told me:

Broken relationship, it knocked me side-ways, I carried on coping and I went through all sorts of emotions. In May I started to feel depressed, by mid June one day it affected me physically and my legs gave way. I was queasy and nauseous. I went to the doctor and he said it was a virus and to come back in a week. I was annoyed with him and chose another doctor. He did blood tests but, again, he said I was fine and nothing was wrong.

I'm tired, I have weak legs, a queasiness feeling and I'm sleepy. I've tried to understand it. I'm very tearful, not really interested in anything. It must be depression. I don't want anti-depressants and I've tried St John's Wort. But I'm not feeling well physically.

I'm so tired and it feels like I'm going down a slippery slope. I had hopes and we talked about marriage. My hopes were bigger than I'd acknowledged. Now there is loss of hopes and loss of friendship. I'm too tired to walk. I forced myself recently and ended up with exhaustion.

It was a shock. I felt destroyed. Something died. Like a murder, I couldn't believe it was happening. I couldn't believe it. I felt so awful. He rang and said we needed to talk. I didn't think anything of it. We went out for dinner. He was saying the words. I wasn't hearing them. He didn't see any future and it would be best to stop. I was crying. I couldn't eat. He got the bill. I couldn't believe it was happening. He said a lot of stuff.

I'm off my food. I'm weak physically. I've become nauseous. I'm burping, like it's getting rid of the tension.

I'm normally really forward and happy on my own. I'm finding it really difficult not feeling well. I'd been on my own for 10 years, then he came in.

Two days after her first dose of Ignatia 200c she said she was feeling a bit better.

She said she had a fear that something drastic would happen, like she'd have a heart attack and nobody would be there. She really wanted to eat and felt better eating in company so she arranged to meet friends for lunch. She also had some other friends over to her house to start a book-reading circle and found that really helpful too.

At her follow-up a month later she'd been out all day, was sighing less and was 'thinking about all sorts of stuff' but not about the boyfriend, which was a big improvement as that was all she could talk about at her first consultation.

When I first saw her she was too ill to leave the house to even do her food shopping and after three doses of Ignatia 200c over 2 months she improved so much she got a part-time job.

So, what is the story behind Ignatia?

It's made from the Ignatius Bean that grows in China and the Philippine Islands. The tree it grows from was named after Saint Ignatius Loyola, the founder of the Jesuit Order, by some of his Spanish Fathers. The herbal use is as a tonic and stimulant similar in action to Nux Vomica and used for 'heart trouble', but it is a highly active and powerful poison.[3]

The ripe, dried seeds are used to make the remedy which was proved by Hahnemann, and the provings revealed it was a 'great nerve remedy'.

So what would be poisonous becomes healing in Homeopathy.

In the Materia Medica we see symptoms such as 'the emotional element is uppermost' and 'effects of grief and worry', and most importantly in my case above, 'Persons mentally and physically exhausted by long concentrated grief'.[4]

On a more general level, there is sighing, refusing to eat and loss of appetite. The things you would expect if something traumatic and unhappy has affected you.

The heart symptoms are interesting because my mother, when she was in her late eighties, got palpitations if something emotional happened like hearing some bad news, but one dose of Ignatia 30c stopped the palpitations in their tracks.

The heart symptoms for Ignatia are: 'Palpitation, esp. at night, while engaged in deep thought, in morning in bed. Stitches in region of heart'. The original medicinal properties of Ignatia were linked with its connection to heart symptoms and its Homeopathic application is for emotional upsetments.

So if you feel despair at a relationship that has ended, or you are suffering from emotional shock and loss, remember Ignatia, the wonderful Homeopathic remedy that will help heal a broken heart.

The following case is an example of treatment that can be given, even if someone is seriously ill. This is not a 'Home Treatment' case, but one that demonstrates how Homeopathy helped someone at the end of their life.

A Case of Apis to Help Nephrotic Syndrome

I am going to tell you about a case I treated, but I will mainly focus on the process I went through while the case progressed. Early in my practice I started a support group for local healers and met a young lady whose mother was terminally ill with nephrotic syndrome. I offered to help because I intuited during a group meditation that her mother wasn't quite ready to leave this world. That intuition served me well, because even though she'd been given 8 months to live, she managed, under constant weekly/fortnightly Homeopathic care, to live another 2½ years. And during that time she set her personal and religious affairs in order and made her peace with her Maker and died when *she* was ready.

When I first took Alice's case in May 2003, I was a bit dismayed at how ill she actually was, how swollen her legs were, and that she was in a lot of pain. I asked her how she was feeling and she replied: 'I'm tired. My mind is willing but my body isn't up for it.'

Her legs were like tree trunks, stiff and full of fluid and she was finding it hard to walk.

She'd seen a kidney specialist in January who said her condition was 'caused' by glomerulonephritis (Bright's disease) and she'd been subjected to ECGs and X-rays and was told she'd lost 50% of her kidney function and was 'losing protein'.

She'd been prescribed diuretic tablets which had reduced her weight from 12¼ stone to 10¼ (172 lb to 144 lb), but she'd had an allergic reaction to them and had come out in a rash 'like stinging nettles' which made her itch and scratch so much she couldn't sleep.

Two of her sons are GPs (she had five children) and 'because of them' she agreed to a kidney biopsy but at the last minute decided against it and the consultant 'blew his top, he was in panic mode' and made her sign a disclaimer, and that was that. She was 'finished with the hospital'.

She then went to see a herbalist, changed her diet to fruit and veg, soups, beans, chicken and cottage cheese. Ten days before, her weight had crept up to 11 stone (154 lb) and she was itching and scratching.

Her symptoms had started in the previous October when she started to have 'frothy urine' and 'swollen feet'. She had been very tired but 'very busy in the allotment' and had been commuting on the train from the West Country to Aberdeen to tend to her ageing parents. Before both her parents died, she had nursed her dad, travelling every 2 weeks to see him and 'got no sleep' and then contracted shingles after he died. I said I'd do my best to reduce the oedema, as that was what was causing the most distress. She loved vinegar and dancing so I prescribed Sepia 30c and said I'd see her again in a month.

I then went off to read up as much as I could about her condition.

Having never treated anyone so ill before, I consulted a Homeopath also trained in medicine and was advised that Solidago was a good remedy to try. I also decided to use the MYMOP (Measure Your Medical Outcome Profile) forms so we could objectively see if she improved.

We got on very well. Alice was a Catholic convert and my mother was the same, so we had a common ground to work on. It was obvious to me that the aggressive and unfeeling treatment she'd had at the local hospital was significant, and the fact that I was prepared to listen to her and how she felt about everything helped pave the way for her to trust me.

The Solidago made no obvious difference to her symptoms and the only remedy that came up the most in articles and repertorisation (analysis with the Repertory: book of Homeopathic symptoms) was Apis. A remedy made from the honey bee.

I gave the first dose of Apis 30c on 25th June. I visited regularly and carried on with the Apis and the main things she reported at these visits were:

- She was reasonable
- Huge amount of wee
- Feeling fine
- Weight now down to 10 stone 3 lb (143 lb)

On 20th October 2003 after an undercurrent prescription of Nat Mur 200c that hadn't done much, I decided to go back to the Apis 30c and said I'd be back the next day, and then a very strange thing happened. Alice said that during the night her throat started to feel funny and at 4am she woke up. Her nose on the left side was 'pouring' like 'water flooding'. She woke again at 5am, 'nose pouring'. She weighed herself and she was 10 stone 2lb. This carried on until my next visit and she felt she had 'got the flu' with her nose 'pouring', sneezing and 'coughing'.

As her kidneys weren't working very well, I viewed this as the only way the extra water in her body (oedema) could be ejected.

By 4th November 2003 her weight was down to less than 10 stone and she was 'weeing like a horse'.

Over the next few months she reported feeling 'fine'. She got a few colds here or there and had a Lycopodium prescription and Sepia, but we seemed to return to Apis as being the most capable of keeping her condition stable.

Most of 2004 was routine and I listened to her make a pilgrimage to Ireland, settle an emotional upsetment with her brother, talk about her mother and her deepest truest feelings. She also went to Paris with her son and had a visit to the seaside. I became a sort of confidante and we built up quite a rapport.

Children Leaving Home

The middle part of Alice's treatment was more of me observing her moods and helping her process how she felt about herself and her family. She even helped me with a proving, as her condition had improved enough for her to get out and about. I asked a more experienced Homeopath to help with the case and we came to a good constitutional.

Eventually all her children left home and when her youngest went to university things seemed to change. In October 2005 she developed breathing problems and this was when I felt the case was beginning to get out of my depth. I took the case to supervision again, but nothing seemed to prevent the inevitable and by Christmas Alice couldn't walk far, her breathing was really bad, and I recommended she visit the local NHS Homeopathic hospital satellite clinic, a suggestion she never took up.

I asked a colleague for input and we changed the prescription to Lycopodium, but Alice wanted to carry on with Apis as it had worked so well in the past.

What could I do? Say 'No'?

Just before Christmas 2005 I arranged to see Alice in the New Year. I needed some time to absorb the huge amount of responsibility that I seemed to have given myself by taking on this case and wanted some time away from the fortnightly visits to 'get myself together'. I was shocked when her husband rang me on the 18th January 2006 to tell me she had died that morning.

Even though we had been working together for over 70 consultations and I knew her condition wasn't easy to treat, I was very sad when Alice died. Her family kindly invited me to the funeral, which certainly helped 'closure'.

I don't think I'd be able to take another case like this one as I spent an enormous amount of time worrying about my prescriptions and worrying about how she was doing. As she got weaker a close friend of hers even emailed me, asking what I was 'doing' to help. This caused me an enormous amount of concern, as I knew she was so well liked, and I had to take that to my supervisor too.

I had heaps of supervision and came to the conclusion that taking a case with serious pathology needs more than one person, and as I'm a lone practitioner, I was glad of the support network I've built up.

I'd learned about every member of Alice's family, even met a few of them, and I felt when she died that I'd lost a member of my own family. Her daughter gave permission for me to write this piece, which feels like saying goodbye to a gentle, kindly aunt.

Chapter Fourteen

Remedies, Where to Get Them, Potencies, Manufacturers, Types of Prescribing

In the UK Homeopathic remedies are available 'over the counter' in some health-food shops and some chemists.

The major manufacturers of remedies are:

- Ainsworths: http://www.ainsworths.com/
- Helios: http://www.helios.co.uk/
- Nelsons: https://www.nelsonspharmacy.com/
  Watch out though as their website is a little confusing and sells supplements and other items, not just Homeopathic remedies.

For a remedy to be Homeopathic, it must have been made in a certain way.

In its most basic form, it must be diluted and succussed. The dilution is easy enough to understand, but the succussion, or 'shaking with impact' of the remedies seems to be completely ignored by people who don't understand Homeopathy.

Hahnemann discovered that the remedies he was using, which were mostly herbs or minerals, worked *better* the more dilute they became. Then he hit on (literally) the idea of increasing the energy in the medicine by shaking the vials and 'striking a hard but elastic item such as a leather-bound book, using an up and down motion of the forearm'.

Thus they were prepared vigorously, not delicately. He called this procedure succussion:

...rubbing a medicinal substance and succussing its solution (*dynamization, potentization*) develops the medicinal powers lying hidden in the medical substance and discloses these powers more and more. The dynamization spiritizes the material substance, if one may use that expression.[1]

The whole procedure to make a Homeopathic remedy is a lengthy and time-intensive practice. What the pharmacists are doing, and Samuel is talking about in this brief quote, is they are filling the remedy with energy. A bit like when you shake a bottle of coke, the energy in the bubbles is released. What he says here is this shaking and banging *increases* the healing powers of the substance. They are 'succussed'. Only a small amount of the procedure can be automated. Most remedies are still made by hand.

Potentised Medicines

Potentised medicines are prepared according to the instructions recorded in the Homeopathic pharmacopoeia. The two main pharmacopoeia used in Europe are the German and French pharmacopoeia, which differ in a number of ways. There is currently a project underway to produce a European Homeopathic Pharmacopoeia to eventually replace the existing ones. Homeopathic medicines are uniquely recognised within the European Union pharmaceutical legislation by two directives (92/73/EEC and 92/74/EEC) which acknowledge the particular nature of Homeopathic medicines and give them special status and requirements alongside the rest of conventional pharmacy.

The main difference in requirements is that for single Homeopathic medicines for which no therapeutic claim is made, proof of efficacy is not required for them to be licensed and be put on the market. There are currently some 3,000+ remedies listed in the Homeopathic Materia Medica. This list is continually being added to, as new medicines are 'proved', i.e. tested, for their therapeutic potential on groups of healthy humans.

Hahnemann actually made the remedies that he dispensed for

his patients himself, rather than using apothecaries, which upset the apothecaries hugely as they were paid by how much product the doctor ordered. This problem still exists today because Homeopathic remedies use such small amounts of substance to get a result and drugs companies are paid by how much and how many of their drugs are sold.

Homeopathic remedies can't be licensed like a branded drug, so no-one can make a fortune out of 'inventing' a remedy. And as each bottle of remedy will cost less than £5 to make, produce and sell at a profit, Homeopaths and Homeopathy are less likely to be influenced by financial considerations and are more likely to be focused on the greater good...

Remember, Samuel only had 50 or so remedies that he used during his lifetime.

Now we have more than 3,000 available, but many of them are what we call 'small remedies' and aren't used much.

The mainstream remedies are the ones that have stood the test of time like Arnica, Aconite and Belladonna and the ones I have suggested in this book.

Potency Scale

Most over-the-counter remedies are made on the centesimal scale. The dilutions are multiples of 100s.

Homeopathic remedies are generally prepared according to one of two scales: the decimal (x) and the centesimal (c).

Dilution and Succussion

In the decimal scale, the dilution factor is 1:10, and in the centesimal scale it is 1:100. Remedies usually have a number, such as 6c or 12x, after their name. This number indicates how many times it has been diluted and succussed, and on which scale; for example, the remedy Arnica 6c has been diluted and succussed six times on the centesimal scale.

More rarely, however, scales such as millesimal (m) and

quinquagintamillesimal (lm) are prepared. According to these scales, remedies are diluted by factors of 1:1,000 and 1:50,000 respectively. The former is used mainly when a single, high-potency dose of a remedy is considered appropriate by the practitioner, while the latter is given when regular gentle dosing is needed in stubborn, chronic cases.[2]

LM potencies are what Hahnemann was experimenting with when he died. These are diluted in a different way.

The LM Potencies

Hahnemann changed the dilution factor from 1:100 to 1:50,000. The 3c trituration powder (details of the preparation of this are in §270) is the starting point for the preparation of the LM scale because all remedies are soluble in water at this point; so any remedy can be utilised, even insoluble materials such as mineral remedies like Aurum that is made from gold.

A grain in weight (0.06gm) of this powder is dissolved in 500 drops (30ml) of 20% alcohol, making a 1:500 dilution of the 0.06gm of 3c, and one drop of this solution is then further diluted in 99 drops of 95% alcohol, filling two thirds of a glass vial, giving a (1 in 500 x 100 = 50,000) solution of the 3c powder. This tube is then succussed 100 times against a firm but elastic object (the famous leather-bound bible) to create the LM 1 medicating liquid.

The LM 1 liquid is then poured onto some poppy-seed granules of which a hundred weigh 1 grain (0.06gm). They are so small that one drop of the alcoholic LM 1 liquid can completely wet at least 500 of them. One granule absorbs at least a 500th of a drop. When this granule is dissolved in a drop of water, and 99 drops of alcohol are added to it, the next LM 2 solution contains a 1/500th x 100 = 1/50,000th of the previous LM 1 liquid. The LM 2 liquid is then succussed 100 times also. The process is continued in this way, simply using the granule as the intermediary to transfer a 500th of a drop instead of the direct addition of a whole drop, as is the case with the centesimal 1:100 ratio.[3]

The benefits of using the LM potency scale is that the patient is less likely to aggravate from the remedy and more likely to recover rapidly and gently.

Retailers

You can easily buy Homeopathic remedies online from these manufacturers.

They all ship worldwide and will quote you by email for any unusual remedies.

- www.helios.co.uk
- www.ainsworths.com
- www.nelsons.co.uk
- www.weleda.co.uk
  This is a small company that produces remedies for Anthroposophic doctors and practitioners and will ship worldwide.

In the USA: http://www.boironusa.com/catalog/single-medicines/

You can buy their products online from Amazon; just search for Boiron in the Amazon search box.

Types of Prescribing*

Just as there are many different ways to make a boiled egg, there are many ways to prescribe and analyse a case. Homeopathy develops according to current needs.

In Hahnemann's day, patients would wait in a waiting room until seeing him. They couldn't make advance appointments, as phones hadn't been invented. Sometimes they would write to him to say they were attending on a certain date, but even that was dependent on modes of transport and weather conditions.

Totality

Hahnemann's main method of prescribing was called The Totality of the Patient.

This took into account all the characteristics of the person, their likes, dislikes, how they responded to weather or certain foods. See Chapter Six, The Whole Person.

This didn't always work so he spent a few more years investigating why he couldn't obtain a total cure for some people. Certain patients got to a better state of health, but no further. Being a persistent person, he investigated why that might be.

Miasmatic Prescribing

However, before he died, he started experimenting with a concept he developed which was based on the idea that some complaints were deeply seated within the human race. An inherited susceptibility.

Through his knowledge of history, he worked out that the first 'complaint' that humans suffered from was 'the itch', which he called 'Psora' and originated as leprosy (now called Hansen's disease).

He wrote about his theories in 1828 in a book called *The Chronic Diseases, Their Peculiar Nature and Their Homoeopathic Cure*:

Psora is that *most ancient, most universal, most destructive,* and yet *most misapprehended* chronic miasmatic disease which for many thousands of years has disfigured and tortured mankind, and which during centuries has become the mother of all thousands of incredibly various (acute and) chronic (non-venereal) diseases, by which the whole civilized human race on the inhabited globe is being more and more afflicted. Psora is the *oldest* miasmatic chronic disease known to us.[4]

His theory was that there were three inherited susceptibilities; the other two he called Syphilis and Sycosis. The former originated from another ancient disease of the same name: syphilis, and the latter from gonorrhoea or 'fig-wart' disease.

In his opus *The Organon* he wrote: 'The True, natural, chronic diseases are those that arise from a chronic miasm.'[5]

So, chronic illness could date back, not just to something that happened in this life, but also to our ancestors. This was quite a profound theory in his time. We don't bat an eyelid to it now and have things like the Human Genome Project that investigated the susceptibility to certain diseases.

So, how does this work in practice?

A Homeopath taking a client's case might notice that a number of family members have all died of the same disease, or been affected by them. In my family my paternal grandfather and great grandfather both died of TB (tuberculosis) and so did my aunt, my father's sister. My older sister's youngest child had a lot of asthma when he was little, which their Homeopath put down to TB running in the family and treated the child with Tuberculinum, the remedy made from diseased tissue from a sufferer of tuberculosis.

Constitutional Prescribing

This is the Homeopathic Holy Grail. To correctly take a case, summarise the client's illness and repertorise (grade the symptoms and analyse the case using the Homeopathic book, the Repertory) the symptoms and give a prescription based on the client's personality. On the 'who' that they are, not the 'what' that they are suffering from. This should, in an ideal world, produce a remedy that mirrors completely the client's constitution. Having been in private practice for over 15 years, I can safely say this doesn't happen all the time. Not all clients are the same, obviously, and people being people in a busy world, don't have the time to explain in great detail exactly everything about themselves.

They might only want one or two symptoms to improve. Or

they might not know how deeply Homeopathy can help, so sometimes part of my job is to *educate* my clients (and I use that word carefully) in Homeopathic philosophy. I do always aim to make a constitutional prescription. That's the best form of prescribing.

As Dr Margaret Tyler, a great constitutional prescriber, said:

> You have to say, not 'this is a case of rheumatism, and I might try Rhus, because Rhus is a very good medicine for rheumatism', but 'this is a Sepia patient, and, whatever ails her, it is Sepia she needs, and no other medicine'. My goodness! If I had known that from the beginning.[6]

When it works, the client not only has their symptoms relieved, but also their life changes completely, for the better. Some clients change jobs, or move house, or get married, or have children, or re-arrange their marriages, get divorced, whatever they need to make their lives more liveable. That's when the remedy has been literally 'life changing'.

But we have to start somewhere, so don't feel bad about using Homeopathic remedies here and there to assist your health particulars. That form of prescribing is what most people are used to, and has a place in health care, just it isn't entirely Homeopathic.

A good constitutional prescription can empower a client to make the personal changes necessary to live a life of freedom from illness.

The Single Remedy versus Multiple Remedies

Some practitioners, especially those in France and other European countries, like to prescribe more than one remedy at a time. You might get one for a headache, one for bad tummy and another to build up your immunity. I don't think Hahnemann ever prescribed like this, so I'm not sure how this method came about. I suppose the idea is at least one of them might work! Which is true, but how will they know which one?

In the single remedy method that Hahnemann aspired to, one remedy was given at a time, until it stopped working. I did that in the case of Alice with the nephrotic syndrome. She had other remedies sometimes to support her, but we kept coming back to Apis as it helped her so much.

Undercurrent Remedies

When treating someone for a condition that is terminal or extremely life threatening, a remedy might be given in high potency to support a certain organ or clear a miasmatic taint, or a past bad experience.

When I was working with the Drug and Alcohol Unit we would sometimes prescribe high-potency Nat Mur if a client had had an extremely unhappy or sad past. Maybe there was some sort of trauma or bullying or sexual abuse and we would start the case by clearing this first.

Another French method of prescribing is to give a remedy to support an organ, maybe the pancreas or the heart, while also giving a constitutional remedy. Again, I don't know if Hahnemann used this method, but it does work in certain cases.

How Often to Repeat the Remedy

This is a constantly asked question by beginning Homeopaths. There are a lot of opinions! My take is, if you're still feeling bad, carry on taking the remedy. If you feel some improvement, then stop.

Unlike conventional medicines, which are prescribed on body weight or in doses to prevent you being poisoned, Homeopathic remedies can't cause you to overdose or have side-effects.

What you are observing and watching out for are signs of improvement. If you take a remedy and feel a bit better, then wait a few hours before you have another dose.

Let me give you an example:

You've got a really bad cold. You're shivery, anxious and feeling horrible. You've decided (correctly!) to take Arsenicum 30c.

You have your first dose on waking, have a small amount of breakfast and then sit around for about an hour feeling wretched.

By mid-morning, your nose is less runny but you're tired of sitting down and can't find any piece of furniture that suits you. You feel a little like Goldilocks and the Three Bears. Nothing fits.

You take another dose and your desire to wander around the house has decreased. You can sit long enough to read a magazine and your pounding headache has lessened slightly. You can manage a drink without having to sip it. These are signs that you are recovering.

By lunchtime you're thinking about having something to eat, which you manage.

By late afternoon you're feeling anxious. You have another dose of 30c and perk up a little.

By bedtime you're over the worst of your cold.

Only YOU can decide if you need more remedy. I can make loads of suggestions, but luckily Homeopathy puts you in the driver's seat and allows you to observe your symptoms and decide yourself how you're feeling. As a complete general rule, you can repeat a low-potency remedy more frequently than a high potency. A 6c three times a day won't push you into aggravation, unless you continue dosing yourself for weeks at a time. But if you're right in the middle of an acute episode of something, you can repeat the remedy every 30 minutes until things settle down.

ALWAYS write down how you feel and keep checking with yourself or your partner or family/friends for feedback. It can sometimes happen that you feel marvellous, but you might be deluded. I certainly wouldn't recommend self-prescribing for serious mental health issues. See a practitioner; you'll need someone unconnected to you to make a correct assessment of your mental state.

Chapter Fifteen

Training

The first book I ever read on Homeopathy was Kent's *Lectures on Homoeopathic Philosophy*. It wasn't exactly a beginner's book on Homeopathy, in fact it was one of the standard texts I later had to learn at college, but it was an inspirational read.

Even though Mr James Tyler Kent was writing about health-related matters from hundreds of years ago, and the language was outdated and very wordy and cumbersome, his excitement and dedication to his craft shone through. Plus, on reading it, I realised a lot of what I thought about health and disease was terribly wrong. Homeopathy seemed to answer a lot of my own health questions and also offered me the new life I eventually lived.

Training in Homeopathy
There are two distinct types of practitioner in the UK:

1. Those that have trained only in Homeopathy
2. Those that have already gained a degree in medicine and taken a postgraduate qualification in Homeopathy

Sometimes the two overlap as you can train with a Homeopathic college if you're a 'medical professional', but you can't train with the medical institutions if you haven't already gained medical qualifications.

The information I've supplied can vary considerably over time, as most organisations are privately owned/run, so I will only mention those that have either existed for a long time, or I have used, or I personally know about.

1. Training only in Homeopathy

In the UK you can practise as a professional Homeopath after a minimum of 4 years' training. You don't need any qualifications to enrol and don't have to be trained in medicine. (See training for medical professionals below.)

All courses include anatomy and physiology, pathology and disease.

Fees vary, but most courses cost around £2,500 to £4,000+ per academic year, depending on final qualification.

http://www.homeopathycollege.org
The Centre for Homeopathic Education offers degree level BSc Hons, also beginner levels and qualifications in-between. Based in Regent's Park in London.

http://www.homeopathyschool.com
The School of Homeopathy is based in Gloucestershire and teaches to diploma level. They offer attendance, correspondence and e-learning.

http://www.hchuk.com
Hahnemann College of Homeopathy offers online courses, attendance courses, all at diploma level. Based in Slough.

http://www.conhom.com
The Contemporary College of Homoeopathy offers levels of training from beginner to professional and provides a licentiate on qualification. Based in Bristol.

2. Training for medical professionals: doctors, dentists, pharmacists and nurses

http://www.facultyofhomeopathy.org
The Faculty was incorporated by an Act of Parliament in 1950 that recognises their role in regulating the education, training

and practice of Homeopathy by the medical profession. They organise training in various locations in the UK.

There is also training available for homeopathic vets:
http://www.bahvs.com/
The British Association of Veterinary Surgeons was founded in 1982 to advance the understanding, knowledge and practice of veterinary Homeopathy. It aims to stimulate professional awareness of Homeopathy and to encourage and provide for the training of veterinary surgeons in the practice of Homeopathy.

First-Aid Training
In the UK first-aid courses are organised by the British Red Cross: http://www.redcross.org.uk/
and St John Ambulance http://www.sja.org.uk/
The training you will need is called 'essential first aid' or 'basic first aid for baby and child' if you're a parent.

Books on Homeopathy
Without doubt, to learn the most about Homeopathy it's best to read 'from the horse's mouth' and get stuck into Hahnemann's *The Organon of the Medical Art*. There are plenty of versions. The cheapest are Indian reprints. You can read most of his books for free at The Internet Archive: www.archive.org where volunteers have scanned them.

Organon of the Medical Art, Dr Samuel Hahnemann, edited and annotated by Wenda Brewster O'Reilly (adapted from the sixth edition 1842); second printing, 1997, Birdcage Books, USA
I think the best translation, as the original was written in German, is by Wenda Brewster O Reilly. Her version is great, as she's spent plenty of time getting the meaning of what Samuel wrote.

Blackie, M. *Classical Homoeopathy*, Beaconsfield Publishers, 1986
— *The Challenge of Homoeopathy*, Unwin Hyman, 1985
Margery Grace Blackie (1898–1981) was an orthodox doctor who became the Homeopath of Queen Elizabeth II. Her writing is accessible and very readable. She also writes from personal experience.

Boericke, W. *Materia Medica with Repertory*, Boericke & Tafel, 1927
This is a 'pocket-sized' Materia Medica, great for checking remedy sources, with a short repertory at the back. Great also for suggestions on potency.

Castro, M. *The Complete Homeopathy Handbook: A Guide to Everyday Health Care*, Macmillan, 1995

Coulter, CR. *Portraits of Homeopathic Medicines*, Volumes 1 & 2, North Atlantic Books, 1986, 1988
Great descriptions of the constitutional remedies. Excellent way to learn about remedy types.

Hahnemann, Samuel. *The Chronic Diseases: Their Peculiar Nature and Their Homoeopathic Cure*, 1845, first English edition, reprint 1998, Homoeopathic Book Service, Sittingbourne, Kent, 2 volumes
It's almost impossible to get an original physical copy of this any more. It comes in two volumes; the first part has his theories of miasms and the second part what he calls his antipsoric medicines. You can find it at the Internet Archive or you might find a reprint from India, but make sure you have the second bit as it lists the actual proving symptoms of the 48 remedies he used.

Iyer, TS. *Beginner's Guide to Homoeopathy (The Stepping Stone to Homoeopathy)* B Jain Publishers Ltd, New Delhi
I was recommended this book by Mike Bridger, a lecturer at my first college, and as he said, it's not exactly a beginner's book as it

includes almost every type of illness, philosophy, materia medica, a summary of the *Organon*, a therapeutic index and more. Great book though and worth having on your Homeopathic shelf.

Kent, JT. *Repertory of the Homoeopathic Materia Medica and a Word Index*, 1897, reprint 1995, B Jain Publishers Ltd, New Delhi
This is the repertory or 'book of symptoms' that most students begin with. It's been modernised, updated and made into computer software, but the book has stood the test of time as being logically arranged from Mind down the body to Generalities.

Kent, JT. *Lectures on Materia Medica*, 1904, reprint 1993, B Jain Publishers Ltd, New Delhi
Mr Kent followed Hahnemann as a leader in Homeopathy and taught and lectured extensively on remedies and philosophy. This book lists in alphabetical order over 200 remedies that Kent delivered at the Post Graduate School of Homoeopathics in the USA. Most copies are now reprints from India.

Kent, JT. *Lectures on Homoeopathic Philosophy*, reprint 1993, B Jain Publishers Ltd, New Delhi
This was the first Homeopathic book I ever read, and it's a fascinating series of lectures that Kent delivered to his students in the late 1890s.

Lessell, CB. *The World Travellers' Manual of Homoeopathy*, CW Daniel Company Ltd, 1993
Fantastic book with lots of information about foreign travel, the sort of injections you will legally need for various countries, and most importantly the sorts of illnesses and diseases you might catch while out there, with suggestions for treatment and remedies.

Lockie, A. *The Family Guide to Homeopathy*, Hamish Hamilton, 1998

Lockie, A, and Geddes, N. *The Complete Guide to Homeopathy*, Dorling Kindersley, 1995

These are wonderful books written by a UK General Practitioner (GP), which include every possible medical condition you can think of with suggestions for remedies to self-prescribe.

Schroyens, F. *Synthesis Repertorium Homoeopathicum*, Homoeopathic Book Publishers, 1995

Enormous book of symptoms, updated with many modern remedies and provings (some of mine are in some editions!). Useful additions are words that are similar and related rubrics, so you can explore a certain symptom in different ways.

Shepherd, D. *Magic of the Minimum Dose*, CW Daniel Company Ltd, 1964
— *A Physician's Posy*
— *Homoeopathy for the First Aider*
— *More Magic of the Minimum Dose*
— *Homeopathy in Epidemic Diseases*

Dr Dorothy Shepherd (1885–1952) was a conventional doctor who trained in Homeopathy. I love all of Dorothy's books; they're written in sensible language, are down to earth and very readable, plus she writes from personal experience.

Speight, Phyllis. *A Study Course in Homoeopathy*, CW Daniel Company Ltd, 1979
— *Tranquillisation the Non-Addictive Way*, CW Daniel Company Ltd, 1990
— *Homoeopathy: A Home Prescriber*, CW Daniel Company Ltd, 1992

Prolific author of numbers of easy-to-read books on Homeopathy aimed at the beginner.

Tyler, ML. *Homoeopathic Drug Pictures*, CW Daniel Company Ltd, 1942

Margaret Lucy Tyler (1875–1943) was an English Homeopathic doctor who was a student of James Tyler Kent. Margaret Tyler became one of the most influential Homeopaths of all time. This book describes the remedies in a more creative way than previous Homeopathic literature and gives a 'personality' to each remedy.

Yasgur, Jay. *Yasgur's Homeopathic Dictionary and Holistic Health Reference*, Van Hoy Publisher, Greenville, Pennsylvania, USA, 1998

Very useful dictionary that helps you make sense of all the old-fashioned words in the classic texts by Kent and Hahnemann.

Glossary

Acute – An illness of sudden onset and short duration.

Aggravations – That which makes the patient's symptoms worse. It is written using the symbol <

It is also a term used to describe when a patient's symptoms get briefly worse as they recover their strength and health.

Ameliorations – That which makes the patient's symptoms better.

It is written using the symbol >

Causation – The 'trigger' that begins an illness, i.e. what brought it on, e.g. getting cold and wet; bad news, suppressed anger.

Chronic – A long-standing and persistent illness that may go unchanged or get progressively worse.

Concomitant – A symptom occurring at the same time as another symptom but not directly related, e.g. 'When I get my headache, my eyes water.'

Generals – Symptoms relating to the whole person; the patient is able to describe them, e.g. 'I feel hot'; 'I feel weak and drowsy'. This will include thirst, sleep, appetite, energy levels.

Materia Medica – A book containing all the remedies listed in alphabetical order, including their origins, how they affect the body from the mind to the feet, with some clinical additions, and generally summarises provers' feedback.

Mental/Emotional – The psychological components of any disease which may be displayed by the patient, e.g. fearful, irritable, and weepy.

Miasm – A philosophical concept that there is an inherited susceptibility to certain disease states. Hahnemann called the ones he referred to as Psora (the itch), Syphilis, Sycosis and Tubercular. Rajan Sankaran has added Ringworm, Malaria, Typhoid, Leprosy and Cancer.

Modalities – Anything which modifies the symptoms, e.g. 'My cough is better lying down'; 'My headache feels worse in a warm, stuffy room'. Modalities are either aggravations or ameliorations.

Mother Tincture – Starting, raw substance that a remedy is made from such as a plant, mineral, or animal product.

Nosode – Remedy made from diseased tissue. For instance Tuberculinum is made from diseased tissue from someone who had tuberculosis. Mainly used in miasmatic prescribing.

Particulars – Symptoms that relate to a part of a person, e.g. 'My throat is painful'.

Potency – This indicates the strength of the remedy which is achieved by dilution from the mother tincture of the original substance. The greater the dilution and succussion, the higher the potency.

Provings – The taking of a Homeopathically potentised substance by a healthy individual which brings out symptoms of the disease which that substance will then cure.

Remedies – Homeopathic medicines made from plant, mineral, animal and imponderable sources. They may be in the form of liquid, pills, powder, granules or ointment. They come in a range of potencies.

Repertory – Book of symptoms. Listed alphabetically, in segments of the body starting from the Mind, to the Generals. Homeopaths use these to look up a patient's symptoms. All the information has been researched from the provers' journals and feedback during the provings.

Rubric – Short keynote or sentence from the Repertory used to describe a remedy and using a summarised version of the provers' exact words.

SAI – Abbreviation for **sensation as if** as expressed by the patient of what it feels like. For example, the patient with a sore throat may tell you that s/he has 'a sensation as if there is a lump in the throat', 'sensation as if there is a tight band around the head'.

SRP – Abbreviation for **strange, rare and peculiar symptoms** not common in the illness and unique to the individual, e.g. thirstlessness with high temperature, chilly but wants to be uncovered.

Succussion – Vigorous shaking of the remedy during its preparation to increase its vibrancy.

Symptoms – Changes in mind and body that the patient is able to describe. They can therefore be subjective but are of great importance because they are what the patient perceives.

References

Introduction

1. *The Family Guide to Homeopathy: The Safe Form of Medicine for the Future*, Dr Andrew Lockie, 1989, Hamish Hamilton Ltd, Penguin Group, London
2. *Organon of the Medical Art*, Samuel Hahnemann, edited by Wenda Brewster O'Reilly, 1996, Birdcage Books, Redmond, Washington, USA

Chapter One

1. *Samuel Hahnemann: The Founder of Homoeopathic Medicine*, Trevor M Cook, 1981, Thorsons Publishers Ltd, Wellingborough, Northamptonshire, p59
2. http://www.parliament.the-stationery-office.co.uk/pa/ld 199900/ldselect/ldsctech/123/12303.htm#note7
3. http://www.homeopathy-ich.org/public-services.html
4. http://hpathy.com/past-present/homeopathic-legal-and-regulatory-practice-in-the-united-states/
5. http://apps.who.int/medicinedocs/en/d/Jh2943e/5.18.html
6. http://www.homeopathy-ecch.org/content/view/16/33/
7. http://www.publications.parliament.uk/pa/ld199900/ldselect/ldsctech/123/12303.htm

Chapter Two

1. http://www.who.int/suggestions/faq/en/index.html
2. *The Oxford Dictionary of Current English*
3. *Organon of the Medical Art*, Samuel Hahnemann, edited by Wenda Brewster O'Reilly, 1996, Birdcage Books, Redmond, Washington, USA
4. *Homeopathy, Healing and You*, Vinton McCabe, 1997, St Martin's Press, New York
5. *Miranda Castro's Homeopathic Guides: Mother and Baby:*

Pregnancy, Birth and Your Baby's First Years, 1996, Pan Books, London

6. http://www.mhra.gov.uk/Safetyinformation/Howwe monitorthesafetyofproducts/Medicines/TheYellowCardSche me/Informationforhealthcareprofessionals/Adversedrugrea ctions/index.htm

7. *Organon of the Medical Art*, Samuel Hahnemann, edited by Wenda Brewster O'Reilly, 1996, Birdcage Books, Redmond, Washington, USA

8. *How We Die*, Sherwin B Nuland, 1997, Vintage Books, Random House, New York

9. *Samuel Hahnemann: The Founder of Homoeopathic Medicine*, Trevor M Cook, 1981, Thorsons Publishers Ltd, Wellingborough, Northamptonshire

10. *Organon of the Medical Art*, Samuel Hahnemann, edited by Wenda Brewster O'Reilly, 1996, Birdcage Books, Redmond, Washington, USA

11. Sad/Happy thoughts research
http://news.bbc.co.uk/1/hi/ health/3198935.stm

Chapter Three

1. *The Dynamics and Methodology of Homeopathic Provings*, Jeremy Sherr, 1994, Dynamis Books, Malvern, UK

2. http://www.homeoint.org/morrell/articles/firstprovings.htm

3. https://www.quintilesclinicaltrials.co.uk/upcoming-trials/

4. http://www.alternative-training.com/docs/SOH/Provings/ Proving_of_Cladonia_Rangiferina.pdf

5. http://archive.today/ZB4oE

Chapter Four

1. *First Aid Homoeopathy in Accidents and Ailments*, DM Gibson MB, BS (Lond.) FRCS (Edin.), FFHom, sixteenth edition, 1993, The British Homoeopathic Association, London

2. http://www.who.int/mediacentre/factsheets/fs310/en/index

2.html

3. *The Only Way to Stop Smoking Permanently*, Allen Carr, 1995, Penguin, London

4. *Treatise on the Effects of Coffee*, Dr Samuel Hahnemann, 1876, AF Worthington and Co.
   https://archive.org/details/treatise oneffec01hahngoog

5. http://www.hassandlass.org.uk/reports/2002data.pdf

Chapter Five

1. http://www.meningitis.org/
   National registered charity, funds research to prevent meningitis and septicaemia and to improve survival rates, offers befriending support and membership to people affected

2. www.stroke.org.uk/
   The Stroke Association is the UK's stroke charity. They support stroke survivors, families and carers, and fund research into the prevention and treatment of stroke.

3. www.bhf.org.uk/
   The British Heart Foundation is a UK heart charity.
   www.heart.org/
   The American Heart Association aims to reduce death caused by heart disease and stroke.

4. www.asthma.org.uk/
   A UK asthma charity
   www.aafa.org/
   FREE information and resources from a national non-profit organisation for people with allergies and asthma

5. *Warning Signs & Similar Symptoms: A Desktop Reference Guide for Alternative and Complementary Practitioners*, Ernest Roberts BA, LCH, RSHom and Juliet Williams MB BS DSH, 1997, Winter Press, London
   Black's Medical Dictionary, edited by G Macpherson, 38th edition, A&C Black Publishers Ltd, London

Chapter Six

1. *Homeopathy in General Practice*, 'Anecdotal but Significant', RAF Jack MB, ChB, FRCGP, FFHom, FBSMDH, edited by Janet Gray MA, MB, BChir, MRCGP, MFHom, DRCOG, 2001, Beaconsfield Publishers Ltd, Bucks, UK

2. *The Homoeopathic Treatment of Eczema*, Robin Logan FSHom, 1998, Beaconsfield Publishers Ltd, Bucks, UK

3. *Homeopathy, Healing and You*, Vinton McCabe, 1997, St Martin's Griffin Press, New York

Chapter Seven

1. http://www.nhs.uk/Conditions/Painkillers-ibuprofen/Pages/Side-effects.aspx
   Allen's Key Notes and Characteristics with Comparisons of Some of the Leading Remedies of the Materia Medica with Nosodes, reprint edition, 1996, B Jain Publishers Ltd, New Delhi, India
   Concordant Materia Medica, Frans Vermeulen, second edition, 1997, Emryss BV Publishers, Haarlem, The Netherlands
   A Modern Herbal, Mrs M Grieve FRHS, edited by Mrs CF Leyel, 1998, Tiger Books Int. plc, Twickenham, UK
   Pocket Manual of Homoeopathic Materia Medica and Repertory, and a Chapter on Rare and Uncommon Remedies, William Boericke MD, reprint edition, 1996, B Jain Publishers Ltd, New Delhi, India

Chapter Nine

1. *The Chronic Diseases and Their Perculiar Nature and Their Homeopathic Cure*, Samuel Hahnamann, 1904, http://www.archive.org/stream/chronicdiseasest00hahniala/chronicdiseasest00hahniala_djvu.txt
   Black's Medical Dictionary
   Pocket Manual of Homoeopathic Materia Medica and Repertory, and a Chapter on Rare and Uncommon Remedies, William Boericke MD, reprint edition, 1996, B Jain Publishers Ltd,

New Delhi, India

Repertory of the Homoeopathic Materia Medica and a Word Index, James Tyler Kent, 1986, Homoeopathic Book Service, London

Chapter Ten

1. *The Twelve Healers and Other Remedies*, Edward Bach MB, BS, MRCS, LRCP, DPH, 1996, CW Daniel Company Ltd, Essex, UK
2. *Organon of the Medical Art*, Dr Samuel Hahnemann, second printing, 1997, edited by Wenda Brewster O'Reilly, Birdcage Books, Redmond, Washington, USA
3. *The Patient, Not the Cure: The Challenge of Homeopathy*, Margery G Blackie, Physician to Her Majesty The Queen, 1976, Macdonald and Co. (Publishers) Ltd, London

Chapter Eleven

1. Bad sleep 'dramatically' alters body
   http://www.bbc.co.uk/ news/health-21572686
2. *Repertory of the Homoeopathic Materia Medica and Word Index*, James Tyler Kent, 1897, reprinted in 1986, Homoeopathic Book Service
   Concordant Materia Medica, Frans Vermeulen, second edition 1997, Emryss BV Publishers, Haarlem, The Netherlands

Chapter Twelve

1. *Organon of the Medical Art*, Samuel Hahnemann, edited by Wenda Brewster O'Reilly, 1996, Birdcage Books, Redmond, Washington, USA
2. *Concordant Materia Medica*, Frans Vermeulen, second revised edition, Emryss BV Publishers, Haarlem, The Netherlands
3. *Materia Medica of the Human Mind*, compiled by Dr ML Agrawal, 1996, eighth edition, Pankaj Publications, Delhi, India

4. *Synthesis, Repertorium Homeopathicum Syntheticum*, Dr Frederik Schroyens, 1997, Homeopathic Book Publishers and Archibel SA, B Jain Publishers Ltd, New Delhi, India

Chapter Thirteen

1. *The Myth of the Chemical Cure: A Critique of Psychiatric Drug Treatment*, Dr Joanna Moncrieff, revised edition, 2009, Palgrave Macmillan
2. 'A Psychological Model of Mental Disorder', Peter Kinderman PhD
    https://ugc.futurelearn.com/uploads/files/a0/e5/a0e57cfe-c51a-41a1-94a5-adacb98ddb90/Harvard_paper_for_mooc. pdf
3. *A Modern Herbal*, Mrs M Grieve FRHS, 1998, Tiger Books Int. plc, Twickenham, UK
4. *Concordant Materia Medica*, Frans Vermeulen, 1997, Emryss BV Publishers, Haarlem, The Netherlands

Chapter Fourteen

1. *Organon of the Medical Art*, Dr Samuel Hahnemann, edited and annotated by Wenda Brewster O'Reilly (adapted from the sixth edition 1842); second printing, 1997, Birdcage Books, Redmond, Washington, USA
2. *The Encyclopedia of Homeopathy*, Dr Andrew Lockie
3. 'Dose, Dilution and the LM Potencies', John Morgan MRPharmS, RSHom
4. *The Chronic Diseases: Their Peculiar Nature and Their Homoeopathic Cure*, Dr Samuel Hahnemann (first published 1828), reprint 1995, B Jain Publishers Ltd, New Delhi, India
5. *Organon of Medicine*, Samuel Hahnemann, reprint 1996, B Jain Publishers Ltd, New Delhi, India
6. 'How Not to Do It', Margaret Tyler
    http://www.homeopathyhome.com/reference/articles/tyler1. shtml
    Further information on different prescribing methods: A

Guide to the Methodologies of Homoeopathy, Ian Watson, 1991, Cutting Edge Publications, Cumbria, UK

Further Reading

Lansky, Amy. *Impossible Cure: The Promise of Homeopathy*, RL Ranch Press, California, 2003

Master, Farokh J. *Lacs in Homeopathy*, Lutra Services BV, Eindhoven, The Netherlands, 2002
Great introduction to the Homeopathic remedies made from all kinds of milks, humans and animal, with proving information and powerpoints.

Roberts, AH. *The Principles and Art of Cure by Homoeopathy*, Homoeopathic Publishing Company, 1936

Sankaran, R. *The Spirit of Homoeopathy*, Homeopathic Medical Publishers, 1999
— *The Substance of Homoeopathy*
— *The Soul of Remedies*
I especially like *The Soul* as Rajan has listed 100 useful remedies and given us the inner feelings of these remedies as constitutional.

Scholten, J. *Homoeopathy and Minerals*, Stichting Alonissos, The Netherlands, 1993
— *Homoeopathy and the Elements*, Stichting Alonissos, The Netherlands, 1996
A new form of classification of the minerals and elements, dividing them into series.

Shore, Jonathan, MD. *Birds: Homeopathic Remedies from the Avian Realm*, Homeopathy West, California, USA, 2004
Very interesting information on the modern provings of bird remedies.

Ullman, D. *Homoeopathy: Medicine for the 21st Century*, Thorsons Publishers Ltd, Northamptonshire, 1989
— *The Consumer's Guide to Homeopathy: The Definitive Resource for Understanding Homeopathic Medicine and Making It Work for You*, Jeremy P Tarcher, Penguin, New York, 1999
— *The Homeopathic Revolution: Why Famous People and Cultural Heroes Choose Homeopathy*, North Atlantic Books, USA, 2008
Dana is a prolific author and blogger and writes in an easy-to-understand way.

Vithoulkas, G. *Homoeopathy: Medicine of the New Man*, Thorsons Publishers Ltd, Northamptonshire, 1985

Whitmount, EC. *The Alchemy of Healing*, North Atlantic Books, 1993

Homeopathy and Animals

Day, C. *The Homoeopathic Treatment of Small Animals: Principles and Practice*, Wigmore Publications Ltd, London, 1984

Hunter, F. *Before the Vet Calls: Homoeopathic First-Aid Treatment for Pets*, 1984, Thorsons Publishers Ltd, Northamptonshire, 1984

Homeopathy for Children

Borland, DM. *Children's Types*, British Homoeopathic Association, 1940

Castro, M. *Homeopathy for Pregnancy, Birth, and Your Baby's First Year*, St Martin's Griffin, 1993
— *Miranda Castro's Homeopathic Guides: Mother and Baby*, Pan, new edition 1996
Miranda is a British Homeopath who now lives in the USA,

teaching and lecturing. Her friendly writing is empathic and based on her private practice and work with colleges.

Herscu, P. *The Homeopathic Treatment of Children*, North Atlantic Books, 1991

Homeopathic First Aid

Gibson, DM. *First Aid Homoeopathy in Accidents and Ailments*, British Homoeopathic Association, 1982

Shepherd, Dorothy. *Homoeopathy for the First Aider, 1945–1992*, CW Daniel Company Ltd, UK

AYNI
BOOKS

"Ayni" is a Quechua word meaning "reciprocity" – sharing, giving and receiving – whatever you give out comes back to you. To be in Ayni is to be in balance, harmony and right relationship with oneself and nature, of which we are all an intrinsic part. Complementary and Alternative approaches to health and well-being essentially follow a holistic model, within which one is given support and encouragement to move towards a state of balance, true health and wholeness, ultimately leading to the awareness of one's unique place in the Universal jigsaw of life – Ayni, in fact.